Essential Statistics for Bioscientists

Essential Statistics for Bioscientists

MOHAMMED MEAH
School of Health, Sport & Bioscience
Biological and Medical Sciences
University of East London
London
UK

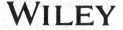

Registered Offices
John Wiley & Sons, Inc., 111 River Street, Hoboken, NJ 07030, USA
John Wiley & Sons Ltd, The Atrium, Southern Gate, Chichester, West Sussex, PO19 8SQ, UK

Editorial Office
9600 Garsington Road, Oxford, OX4 2DQ, UK

For details of our global editorial offices, customer services, and more information about Wiley products visit us at www.wiley.com.

Wiley also publishes its books in a variety of electronic formats and by print-on-demand. Some content that appears in standard print versions of this book may not be available in other formats.

Library of Congress Cataloging-in-Publication Data
Names: Meah, M. S. (Mohammed Shahabu), author.
Title: Essential statistics for bioscientists / Mohammed Meah.
Description: Hoboken, NJ : John Wiley & Sons Ltd, 2022. | Includes bibliographical references.
Identifiers: LCCN 2021060393 (print) | LCCN 2021060394 (ebook) | ISBN 9781119712008
    (paperback) | ISBN 9781119712015 (pdf) | ISBN 9781119712022 (epub)
Subjects: LCSH: Biometry. | Life sciences--Research--Methodology.
Classification: LCC QH323.5 .M43 2022 (print) | LCC QH323.5
    (ebook) | DDC 570.1/5195--dc23/eng/20220202
LC record available at https://lccn.loc.gov/2021060393
LC ebook record available at https://lccn.loc.gov/2021060394

Cover image: © Peter Hermes Furian/Shutterstock, Courtesy of Mohammed Meah
Cover design by Wiley

Set in 10/12pt STIXTwoText by Integra Software Services Pvt. Ltd, Pondicherry, India

SKY10034858_062822

Contents

Acknowledgements

I would like to thank my daughters (Maryam and Zaynah) for their constant encouragement and support during the writing of this book. I would like to thank the many project students over the years whose research project ideas have challenged me to delve into statistics. I have to say a special thank you to my mother (BR Chowdhury) and father (MM Chowdhury) for always being positive and supportive. Many thanks to my colleagues (Rane and Elizabeth) for their insightful comments and suggestions.

Lastly, I would like to thank Wiley Publishers for their encouragement and above all patience and understanding in the completion of this book.

> "If it's green or wriggles, it's biology. If it stinks, it's chemistry. If it doesn't work, it's physics or engineering. If it's green and wiggles and stinks and still doesn't work, it's psychology. If it's incomprehensible, it's mathematics. If it puts you to sleep, it's statistics."
> — *Anonymous*

List of Worked Examples of Statistical Tests

Example	Name	Page	Software
36	Example 6.9: Plotting a pie chart using Microsoft Excel:		EXCEL
37	Example 6.10: Plotting a frequency distribution curve with Excel		EXCEL
38	Example 6.11: How to do a paired t-test		EXCEL
39	Example 6.12: How to do an unpaired (independent) t-test and F test		EXCEL
40	Example 6.13: How to do One-way ANOVA		EXCEL
41	Example 6.14: Bonferroni Post hoc test		EXCEL
42	Example 6.15: How to do 2-way ANOVA		EXCEL
43	Example 7.1: Inputting data and replicates into Prism		Prism
44	Example 7.2: Inputting calculated means, SEMs or SD data into prism		Prism
45	Example 7.3: Calculating the mean, SD and SEM in prism.		Prism
46	Example 7.4: Plotting a histogram in prism		Prism
47	Example 7.5: Producing a cumulative frequency plot using prism		Prism
48	Example 7.6: To determine the correlation coefficient using prism		Prism
49	Example 7.7: Linear regression using prism		Prism
50	Example 7.8: Students t-test using prism		Prism
51	Example 7.9: Paired t test in prism		Prism
52	Example 7.10: One-way ANOVA using prism		Prism
53	Example 7.11: 2-way ANOVA using means		Prism

Example	Name	Page	Software
54	Example 7.12: 2 Way ANOVA with raw data		Prism
55	Example 7.13: Wilcoxon non-parametric test		Prism
56	Example 7.14: Mann-Whitney non-parametric test		Prism
57	Example 8.1: Descriptive stats, graphical display of data, histograms, test of normality		SPSS
58	Example 8.2: Unpaired t test using SPSS		SPSS
59	Example 8.3: To test whether there is a difference between the means of 2 sets of paired measurements.		SPSS
60	Example 8.4: Association between data- correlation		SPSS
61	Example 8.5: Repeated Measures ANOVA		SPSS
62	Example 8.6: One-way ANOVA		SPSS
63	Example 8.7: Two-way ANOVA		SPSS
64	Example 8.8: Wilcoxon test		SPSS
65	Example 8.9: Mann-Whitney test		SPSS
66	Example 8.10: Kruskall Wallis Test (nonparametric one- way ANOVA)		SPSS
67	Example 8.11: Friedman Test (nonparametric repeated measures ANOVA)		SPSS

Introduction

"All life is an experiment. The more experiments you make, the better."

Ralph Waldo Emerson
(1803–1882) - American lecturer, philosopher and poet

The word statistics is derived from the Latin word 'status' – meaning political state or a government. Statistics deals with collection, organization, presentation, analysis and interpretation of data to obtain meaningful and useful information. Statistics can be split into two major areas, namely, descriptive and inferential. Descriptive statistics involves collecting, summarizing, and presenting data. Inferential statistics involves analysing sample data to draw conclusions about a population.

Statistics is an area which is often much reduced in the curriculum of undergraduate bioscience degree courses. Statistics tends to be linked to research modules. Lecturers often assume that students have a strong grasp of mathematical and statistical concepts including data analysis. However, the reality is that most students are 'rusty' in these areas, particularly in statistics. The most urgent need for statistics is usually for the research project which is typically in the final year of the undergraduate degree (level 6). It is unclear, during undergraduate studies, how much and when statistics should be taught. In addition, there are a variety of software packages which can be used to perform statistical analysis, and display data, not all of which can be accessed or used competently by the students. Indeed, it would be fair to say that existing software can produce extensive statistical analysis, but choosing an appropriate test and interpreting the data analysis can be challenging. It is rare to have the luxury to be able to consult a resident statistician in the Bioscience Department.

There are a variety of statistical software packages, which vary in the difficulty of use, and in what tests they can perform. An additional bonus is the ability to plot graphically, mean and individual data. The most popular software packages used currently to perform statistics and present data in graphical form are **Excel (Microsoft), Prism (GraphPad) and SPSS (IBM)**. Microsoft Excel is a popular spreadsheet software package which is easily available, easy to use for data analysis (although types of analysis are limited), and useful to plot data graphically (limited in detail of graph). Prism is good for statistical analysis but excellent for plotting data (graphs produced are of professional standard). SPSS is the most complex, but most comprehensive statistical package. It allows a very detailed analysis of data using a wide range of tests. However, it is weak in interpreting the statistical analysis and the level of detail in plotting graphs.

A core module that most students would do is a research project. This requires them to put forward a research proposal, in which they design experiments and formulate hypotheses, collect data, analyse data, and then write a research report. From my many years of supervising undergraduates and postgraduate projects, I have observed that firstly, narrowing a project down to a specific aim and secondly, applying statistical analysis to the data obtained causes the most anxiety in students.

Essential Statistics for Bioscientists, First Edition. Mohammed Meah.
© 2022 John Wiley & Sons Ltd. Published 2022 by John Wiley & Sons Ltd.

Having taught bioscience students for more than 25 years, I am clear that more help, guidance and resources should be made available to students in using statistics and displaying data. This book is intended for all undergraduate students at levels four (year 1), five (year 2) and six (year 3), studying the biological sciences (biomedical science, medical physiology, pharmacology, pharmaceutical science, human biology, biochemistry, microbiology, and biotechnology). Although most examples are drawn from the biological sciences, the statistical methods and tests covered in the book are applicable and useful for (i) students in other disciplines in medical and health subjects, including medicine, physiotherapy, podiatry, nursing, pharmacy, dentistry, and sports science, (ii) postgraduate research, and (iii) a quick refresher for those who are rusty on statistics and using statistics software.

The book starts from a basic level and builds in complexity, allowing readers to dip into the area they are more familiar with. It does not assume any prior knowledge of the area. The book layout is as follows:

Chapter 1	introduces common terms used in statistics
Chapter 2	shows an overview of how to display data
Chapter 3	considers statistical significance and choosing inferential tests
Chapter 4	gives background to some common parametric tests
Chapter 5	gives background to some common nonparametric tests
Chapter 6	explains how to use Microsoft Excel with examples
Chapter 7	explains how to use GraphPad Prism with examples
Chapter 8	explains how to use IBM SPSS with examples
Chapter 9	briefly considers misinterpretations/errors of statistics in analysis.

The appendices have sections on common formulas and symbols, deciding on sample size, historical milestones in statistics, background to Prism, answers to sample problems, and reference tables of critical values for statistical tests.

This book is not comprehensive in its coverage (the focus is on the most commonly used statistical tests in biomedical science) as that would have increased the size and complexity of the book. I have tried to keep the mathematical input to a minimum; however, there are areas such as analysis of variance where this was unavoidable. For those who want more depth and detail in maths and statistics, suggestions for further reading are provided. This book does not cover qualitative analysis (e.g. interviewee responses, social context, interactions with people).

This book:

1. Introduces statistical terms and analysis from the basics to a more advanced level.
2. Shows clear step by step use of three common software used in analysing data and producing graphs.
3. Uses examples of common statistical tests.
4. Does not describe areas such as enzyme and substrate reactions (e.g. Scatchard plots), or non-linear curve fitting or multiple regression.
5. Helps in deciding the factors to consider for study designs.
6. Helps in choosing appropriate tests to analyse data and to display data.

The reader should be able to answer the following questions from the use of this book.

What:

- Is your study design?
- Sample size is appropriate?
- Are the descriptive statistics appropriate for the sample data?
- Is the difference between standard deviation and standard error of the mean?
- Is a confidence interval?
- Is a normal distribution?
- Is significance and how do you test for it?
- Is the interquartile range?
- Is the difference between parametric and non-parametric tests?

How do you:

- Graphically describe your data?
- Plot a frequency distribution plot?
- Check if the sample data is normally distributed?
- Decide on which statistical test to use?
- Do a paired (related groups) t test?
- Do an unpaired (independent groups) t test?
- Do a non-parametric test (Wilcoxon)?
- Do a non-parametric test (Mann–Whitney)?
- Do a 1-way ANOVA test?
- Do a repeated measures 1-way ANOVA?
- Do a 2-way ANOVA test?
- Do a correlation test?
- Use Microsoft Excel software to do statistical analysis?
- Use SPSS software to do statistical analysis?
- Use Prism software to do statistical analysis?

I hope the readers and users of this book will (a) get a better understanding of statistical concepts and (b) be able to use the software packages with more confidence and thereby aid them in their degree studies.

Mohammed Meah BSc MSc PhD FHEA
Senior Lecturer in Physiology
Course Leader for Medical Physiology
and Human Biology
University of East London,
London

> **"It would be so nice if something made sense for a change."** *Lewis Carroll (1832–1898), English novelist. From the book Alice in Wonderland*

CHAPTER 1

Basic Statistics

"The word 'statistic' is derived from the Latin status, which, in the middle ages, had become to mean 'state' in the political sense. 'Statistics', therefore, originally denoted inquiries into the condition of a state."

— Wynnard Hooper (1854–1935) - English author

Expected Learning Outcomes

- Explain the common terms used in statistics.
- Describe, interpret and calculate descriptive statistics.
- Distinguish the differences between confidence interval, standard error and standard deviation.
- Outline common study designs.
- Describe the parts of a research proposal.

Data

- Without data there would be no statistics!
- Data is Information that can be analysed, interpreted and presented statistically.
- Data can take many forms, digital data, personal data, sample data, laboratory experimental data, field data, population data.
- In statistics we categorize these into numerical and non-numerical data.

What is Statistics?

The earliest use of statistics came from rulers and governments, who wanted information (**data**), such as the number of people, resources (e.g. food, gold, land) in order to set taxes, fund infrastructure (building projects), raise and maintain armies, and go to war (Appendix 1). To make accurate decisions, ideally you would want to

Essential Statistics for Biocientists, First Edition. Mohammed Meah.
© 2022 John Wiley & Sons Ltd. Published 2022 by John Wiley & Sons Ltd.

collect all the information or data available about a defined group or category. This is called the **population** (the entire group of individuals or observations).

The modern equivalent of this is called a census or survey of the population (usually every 10 years) of a country, which collects information such as the total number of people, ethnicity, age, and gender. The data obtained is called the population data. Some examples include, those with a disease or condition (e.g. diabetes or hypertension), smoking, animals, or plants.

However, it is not practical or possible to get the population data most of the time, so we take a random sample which can be representative of the population. The **sample** is a defined group of individuals or observations such as smoking habits taken from an identified and specific population. The sample should be representative of the population and is chosen by setting inclusion and exclusion criteria. These criteria define the characteristics or features of the sample. For example, inclusion criteria could be healthy, males, aged 20–30; exclusion criteria participants (or subjects) not suitable for selection might be smokers, not on any medication or have a medical condition.

Statistics can also be defined as: a branch of mathematics which involves data collection, data presentation, data analysis, and interpretation of data which comes from a population or sample of the population. In statistics, we usually take data from population samples. A **population sample** consists of a certain proportion/percentage of the total population determined by the researcher. The bigger and

> "By a small sample, we may judge of the whole piece."
> *Miguel de Cervantes (1547–1616), from his novel "Don Quixote"; Spanish novelist, poet and playwright*

more representative the sample size, the more valid would be the results of data analysis. For example, we take height measurements (an example of data collection) of 50 male and 50 female level 5 bioscience students. This sample of 100 students would be taken from a total population of 645 level 5 bioscience students, to determine the average (mean) height of both male and female students. We would then see whether this average height is representative of the average height of all the level 5 bioscience students.

Types of Statistical Methods

In statistics, we analyse sample data to make predictions and generalisations about the population data. The sample data collected is described according to the amount of data (total data), centre of data (average, middle and most commonly occurring) and spread of data (e.g. lowest value and highest value). These are described numerically and called **descriptive statistics**. The statistical terms used in descriptive statistics (e.g. mean, mode, median, standard deviations) are described below.

The statistical terms used in descriptive statistics using a variety of graphs (Chapter 2), this is called **exploratory statistics**. Further analysis to look for differences between sample data and population data, differences between two or more groups of sample data, or looking for associations or relationships between sample groups is called **inferential statistics.** The types of inferential statistical tests used will be determined by data size, data distribution, data type and number of groups of data. Inferential tests can be classified into two types: **parametric** or tests which are based on known probability **distributions** of the population (Chapters 3 and 4), and **non-parametric** which do not follow a distribution (Chapters 3 and 5). A distribution in statistics describes the possible values and likely occurrences of these values (e.g. in tossing a coin, getting a head or tail, and the likelihood of getting heads or tails with further attempts) in experiments (Chapter 2).

Types of Data

Data can be observations or measurements. Data can be classified into **quantitative** (numerical – numbers) or **qualitative** (categorical – non-numerical).

Quantitative Data

This numerical data is split into continuous (lots of data collected in very small steps), and discrete (number of specific events occurring). **Discrete data** take specific number values (e.g. number of pregnancies, number of vaccinations) and give less information. **Continuous data** (e.g. height, weight, cholesterol, cell counts, concentration of substances in fluids, decimals, percentages, ratios) – very small steps, give more information; this type of data are used mainly in parametric tests (Chapter 4).

Qualitative Data

This non-numerical data can be split into **discontinuous data**, such as whole numbers, ranks, scales, gender, colours, species, classes, position in a race, and blood groups. This is also called **categorical data**, which can also be divided into **nominal data** (data which cannot be ranked in size, e.g. blood groups, gender, ethnicity) and **ordinal data** (data which can be ranked, e.g. position in a race, anxiety scale, pain scale, intensity of exercise). This type is predominantly used in non-parametric tests (Chapter 5).

Both quantitative and qualitative data can be expressed by the term **variable**. A variable is a specific factor, property, or characteristic of a population or a sample. It is the name given to the data that is collected, e.g. height, weight, gender, colour, and size.

Collection of Data

Data can be collected from observations (e.g. epidemiological study), surveys (e.g. questionnaires and interviews) or experiments (e.g. clinical trials, pilot study).

Framingham Heart Study (1948)

This was a famous medically important long term epidemiological study, initiated by the National Institute of Health (NIH). It collected a large amount of data on the epidemiology and risk factors of cardiovascular disease in 5209 adults in 1948. They identified hypertension (elevated blood pressure), high cholesterol (fat) levels, and cigarette smoking, as major risk factors for cardiovascular disease (Mahmood *et al.* (2014)).

Surveys

Ask a series of questions where the answers are subjective (based on personal opinion). These can be non-numerical or numerical by adding a number scale to the responses

e.g. (i) anxiety or pain – could be classified into none, mild, moderate, or severe

(ii) Likert Scale – agree, disagree, neither agree or disagree, strongly agree, e.g. module evaluation or describing a product you have bought

(iii) Visual Analogue Scale – an increasing number scale (e.g. 1 is low and 10 is high). An example of this is the Borg Rate of Perceived Exertion which scales the intensity of exercise.

Clinical Trial

A clinical trial compares the effect of one treatment with another. It involves patients, healthy people, or both in four stages (Phase 1 to Phase 4).

The rapid increase in infections and mortality caused by the coronavirus (Covid-19) worldwide in 2019 led to the need to develop effective vaccines. The two most popular vaccines in the UK are the Oxford–AstraZeneca and the Pfizer Biontech. Both of these underwent clinical trials after ethical approval. Each trial involved two groups, in which half the volunteers were given the vaccine and the other half were given a placebo. The groups were randomly selected and were matched (e.g. for age and gender). Volunteers did not know whether they were receiving the vaccine or the placebo, nor did the researchers know (double blind). Prior to using human volunteers, the vaccines were tested on animals.

The Oxford–AstraZeneca trial sampled 23,848 people across the UK, Brazil and South Africa between April and November 2020.

The Pfizer Biontech trial sampled 46,331 people from 153 sites around the world between July and December 2020.

Observations, hypotheses, theories

Before the 20th century, science was based on induction from observations from which theories were formed (e.g. Newton's laws of motion in 1664). Karl Popper, a philosopher in 1935, suggested that theories and laws should be put first as a hypothesis, which would then be tested by experimental hypothesis falsified by observations and experiments (e.g. Darwin's theory of evolution in 1859).

Experiments

An **experiment or study** gathers data from a sample (assumed to be drawn randomly from the population). Experiments test a hypothesis (or prediction) of something happening. For example, suppose you wanted to know if there was a difference between an old treatment and a new treatment for a disease condition. Two predictions which we can make about this are: (i) there will be no difference between the old treatment and the new treatment (called the **null hypothesis**) on the disease condition, or (ii) there will be a difference between the old and new treatments (called the **alternative hypothesis**) on the disease condition.

In experiments, two groups of variables need to be identified. One group is the **dependent variables,** which are the outcome measures of the experiment (e.g. cell size, rate of growth, and cholesterol levels). The other group is the **independent variables,** which are the variables being manipulated in the experiment (e.g. type of treatment (drug, surgery), type of activity (exercise, training) and type of nutrient (protein, vitamin)).

Research Proposal

The experiment could be part of a **research project** (a short- or long-term study), and can be done in the laboratory or field (natural environment). In starting a research project or applying for research funding, it is common to write a **research proposal.** The proposal describes the subject area of the research and has various parts which answer the following questions:

- What is the research area of interest and justification for doing the research?
- What is the aim of the research?
- How will the aim be investigated?
- What are the expected outcomes?

Parts of a Research Proposal

1. **Background literature search**: to see what is known, what is unknown, and whether this study has been done before. This would involve doing literature searches, using key words from the title of the project and **databases** (e.g. in

> "The formulation of the problem is often more essential than its solution, which may be merely a matter of mathematical or experimental skill."
> -*Albert Einstein (1879–1955) - Physicist*

bioscience the most popular are PubMed, Science Direct, Google Scholar), reading primary sources (e.g. journal papers) and secondary sources (e.g. textbooks). It is very important to identify what is unknown or controversial, or where there is a gap of knowledge from previous studies, an observation, or initial investigation (pilot study). This would then be the basis of the rationale (reason) for doing the study. For example, suppose you were interested in doing a research project on exercise training and haemoglobin levels. You would do a literature search with your key words being exercise, training, and haemoglobin. Your search may produce a large number of studies, which you will then need to filter, e.g. human studies, type of exercise, duration of training, gender, year of publication. You then need to identify gaps in knowledge or controversy, i.e. levels of haemoglobin between gender, ethnicity, types, and duration of exercise training.

2. **A clear aim**: typically, this would be a question you want to answer based on the unknown or controversy identified in the background literature search. Ideally, you would want to state a narrow aim (say in the form of a question). For our example, suppose you found in the literature a controversy about the duration of exercise affecting the levels of haemoglobin. Some studies showed there was a difference after three weeks and others showed that the difference was only found after six weeks. You could have an aim such as: Is there a difference in haemoglobin levels after three and six weeks of aerobic exercise training?

3. **Hypothesis**: a prediction of outcomes. This is stated as two parts:

    i. Null hypothesis: there is no difference (in the mean variables) between the control and experimental conditions. For our example, the null hypothesis would be 'there is no difference in mean haemoglobin levels after three and six weeks of training'.

    ii. Alternative hypothesis: there is a difference (in the mean variables) between the control and experimental conditions: 'there is a difference in mean haemoglobin levels after three and six weeks of training'.

4. **Methodology**: methods used to investigate the aim. There are four major parts in methods. An outline of the subjects (human or animal or material), equipment/techniques used, protocol (procedures or steps of the experiment), and analysis of data (statistical tests to be used). These parts would incorporate the following:

    i. Health and safety issues (for the researchers, participants, environment).

    ii. Ethical considerations (e.g. using humans or animals for data collection in the study/experiment).

    iii. How large should the sample size be?

    iv. How many replicates (repeat measurements)?

    v. What are the dependent and independent variables? Independent variables are those being manipulated in experiments and dependent variables are those we measure to see the effect of the manipulation.

    vi. How do you exclude confounding variables (factors that could adversely affect an experiment or other data collection procedure)?

    vii. Control and experimental conditions (what is the baseline or reference and the interventions?)

    viii. Analysis of results (descriptive and inferential statistics).

    ix. Precautions (to ensure you collect relevant study data).

Example of Biomedical experiment methodology

Consider our example: an experiment investigating the effect of exercise training on haemoglobin levels in a group of healthy adults

    i. Health and safety issues (for the researchers, participants, environment): taking blood, preventing infections, laboratory safety, disposal of used materials, e.g. needles, equipment safety will depend on type of equipment used (e.g. cycle ergometer, treadmill), injury during training, first aider availability.

ii. Ethical considerations (e.g. using humans or animals for data collection in the study/experiment): ethics application to Ethics Committee for approval.
iii. How large the sample size should be: depends on the power of experiment required, calculation of sample size.
iv. How many replicates (repeat measurements): depends on protocol and study design, e.g. could have two groups (one group does no training, one does training for six weeks, measure haemoglobin at the beginning and then week by week in both groups). Also measure blood pressure and heart rate to monitor training intensity.
v.   What are the dependent and independent variables (variables being manipulated in experiment are independent variables and dependent variables are the variable we measure to see the effect of the manipulation): dependent variable would be haemoglobin levels, independent variable would be exercise training duration.
vi. How do you exclude confounding variables (factors that could adversely affect an experiment or other data collection procedure): environmental temperature constancy, pressure kept constant, time and day for experiment consistent, stronger design of experiment, e.g. matching subjects.
vii. Control and experimental conditions: this depends on the design, so no training for controls and training for experimental group. The two groups would be matched for state of health, fitness, and age.
viii. Analysis of results: differences in mean haemoglobin levels between controls and experimental group would be tested using an independent t-test.
ix. Precautions: subjects familiar with protocol, i.e. procedures, use of equipment, calibration of equipment, questionnaires to monitor food and fluid intake.

5. **Expected Results:** making predictions on outcomes based on existing literature and the proposal design.
6. **Costs**: of materials, consumables, equipment, animals, facilities, payments for volunteers, and investigators.
7. **Timeline**: breakdown of when various parts of the project will be completed typically as a **Gantt chart** (tabular display of breakdown of the project into various parts and associated timelines to completion of the parts (Figure 1.1)).

As you can see in the Gantt chart below, an estimate has been made of the time allocated to complete the research proposal, ethics application, learn and practice the protocol, collect data, analyse the results, and finally submit the final research

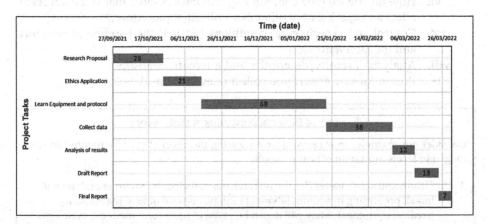

FIGURE 1.1 Gantt chart of research project tasks versus time (days).

report. The times may need to be altered due to problems encountered in the project, e.g. equipment and technique failure, availability of materials, volunteers and funding, and even unforeseen circumstances such as corona virus infections preventing research.

Deciding on the Research Experiment

To investigate the aim of the research and test the hypothesis, one or more experiments are needed. The effectiveness of experiments depends on several factors, including experimental design, sample size, and the statistical tests used for analysis.

Experimental Design   It is crucial to think of the design of the experiment as this will determine whether the aim can be answered, and the type of statistical test you will be using to analyse your results (Chapter 3). How do you decide on the design? There are well known established designs (see section below on study design) which could fit your study.

Steps in choosing the design

Step 1: What is (are) the aim (aims) of your study? The clearer this is, the better, particularly if you can reduce the aim to a specific question.

Step 2: What will you be measuring (what variables) to see an effect, e.g. size, growth, symptoms, heart rate, cholesterol, absorbance?

Step 3: How will you measure your variables? What equipment or techniques and materials will you use?

Step 4: What will you be altering, or manipulating, or intervening (e.g. treatment, training, stress, concentration, dose of drug, vaccines, temperature)? So, you want to know the effect of this change on the measured variable.

Step 5: How many groups will there be, and how do you assign groups (see study designs below)? If you have one group, are they going to act as their own control, and then measure them again following the intervention? You might have two or more separate groups not related to each other.

Step 6: Design the protocol so that errors are reduced, by minimizing all the factors that could affect the experiment (e.g. environment, time of day, temperature, within subject factors (e.g. relaxed or not), between subject factors (type, age, gender, health).

Step 7: If possible, keep your design simple, and ask if it will allow you to collect data that may answer your aim. If your study doesn't fit the well-known study designs or has a complex design, then you may need further advice from your research supervisor or statistician.

Step 8: What analysis will you do: e.g. descriptive statistics, plot graphs, inferential tests to look for differences or associations in the means?

To illustrate the above steps in the design of a study, consider the biomedical study in the text box below.

An example of a biomedical study

Step 1: What is (are) the aim/aims of your study? The effect of arm exercise induced muscle soreness on creatine kinase levels in fit and unfit healthy adults.

Step 2: What will you be measuring (what are the dependent variables)? Creatine kinase (a quantitative marker of muscle damage), soreness scores (subjective scale of soreness).

Step 3: How will you measure your variables? Creatine kinase measured from 20 μL of blood from the finger and blood analyser (Reflotron); Visual Analogue Scale (0 for no soreness to 10 for severe soreness).

Step 4: What will you be altering or manipulating or intervening (independent variables)? Exercise of the upper arms (biceps contraction and relaxation).

Step 5: How many groups will there be, and how do you assign groups? Two groups of 10 healthy subjects, matched for age (age range 18–25 years) and fitness, of any gender. A fitness test on a treadmill (measurement of maximal oxygen uptake, the higher the value, the fitter you are) will be used to split volunteers into fit and unfit groups.

Step 6: What is the protocol? A week before the experiment, volunteers will have their fitness assessed by having their oxygen levels measured (using a metabolic analyser: Cosmed K5) whilst running to exhaustion (speed increased by 1 km hr^{-1} every minute) on a treadmill (Cosmed Mercury). They will then be split into two groups based on their maximal oxygen consumption ($VO2_{max}$), group A (fit) and group B (unfit). One week later, both groups will have their creatine kinase and soreness level measured at rest (control condition). Then they will perform arm exercise (biceps curl) at an intensity of 50% of their maximum in the standing posture until exhaustion. Creatine kinase and soreness levels will be measured at the end of the exercise and 30 minutes after exercise.

Precautions: No food 1 hour before the test, volunteers will be familiarized with the procedures; volunteers will do warm up exercise for 4 minutes at low intensity for both treadmill and arm exercise; safety procedures will be followed for use of equipment and taking blood samples.

Step 7: What is your design? Matched pairs design (groups have been matched for fitness).

Step 8: What analysis will be done? Descriptive statistics (N, mean, SEM, SD) will be calculated using Microsoft Excel. Mean creatine kinase and soreness levels will be plotted against conditions (control, exercise, recovery). Diferences in mean creatine kinase between the fit and unfit groups will be compared using one-way ANOVA (analysis of variance), with significance set at the 95% level ($P < 0.05$).

Note: Prior to developing the study aim, you would have researched the literature for the background and rationale, e.g. muscle soreness, a characteristic pain associated with exercise induced muscle damage (EIMD) in eccentric elbow flexor exercise that has a delayed onset. There is controversy about the levels of EIMD in trained and untrained subjects, and the levels of serum creatine released.

Having obtained an idea about the steps in choosing a study design, let us consider some additional factors to take into consideration in the study design.

Additional Factors to Consider in Deciding the Study Design

i.   Control for the experiment: the baseline to which the intervention in the experiment will be compared to. Will one control be enough, or do you need more (e.g. positive and negative controls)?

ii. Intervention/ manipulation/ treatment: this is the input you are using to see if there is any effect.

iii. Type of sample, e.g. humans, animals, cells.

iv. If using humans: do not inform the subject about intervention (blind), i.e. subject does not know whether receiving placebo (looks like the treatment but lacks active ingredient or effect) or treatment.

v.   Putting groups of subjects with similar characteristics together in a block.

vi. Subjects put into blocks by random selection: randomized experimental design.

vii. Controlled design: subjects carefully chosen.

viii. Replication: repetition of an experiment.

ix. Large enough sample size.

> **"If your experiment needs statistics, you ought to have done a better experiment."**
> *Ernest Rutherford (1871–1937), 1st Baron Rutherford of Nelson, New Zealand - born physicist*

We will now expand on the most important areas, namely controls, sample size, repeating experiments, and common study designs.

Controls   Essential in the study design of any experiment is deciding on a control condition or group. The control group receives no treatment or receives the standard treatment. It is this group which is compared to the experimental or intervention group. The control is the baseline for comparing any changes caused by the intervention or experiment.

There are different types of controls: positive, negative, and blank. A positive control shows the expected result; they would receive an intervention where the expected result is known and would not receive the experimental intervention. A negative control shows the expected result does not occur, so the group or condition would receive something to show no response (e.g. placebo such as a sugar pill in place of the drug), and would not receive the experimental intervention. Sometimes a blank control (which does not have the substance you are testing for, e.g. distilled water) is used (particularly in calibrating instruments and dealing with solutions), before and after an experiment to check the baseline or standard condition.

An assay is a biological method to estimate the concentration of a substance (e.g. protein). A microbiological assay might compare the inhibition of microorganism growth by an antibiotic compared to concentrations of standard antibiotics. Thus, our main experiment is to treat the bacteria with the new antibiotic. Our negative control is treating with a non-antibiotic. Our positive control is to use a well-known established antibiotic.

There are different types of assay methods. One popular method is called ELISA (enzyme-linked immunosorbent assay) which is used to measure hormones (e.g. cortisol) or cytokines which are a variety of small proteins important in cell signalling, immunity and inflammation (e.g. IL6). The concentrations of these substances are very small (e.g. nanograms and picograms per ml). In this method, the positive control is a soluble sample containing the protein; the negative control is the soluble sample which does not have the protein, and a standard sample that has known concentration of the protein.

Sample Size for Studies   Before an experiment is carried out it is useful to calculate the power of the experiment. The **power** is the probability (likelihood of an event occurring) that an experiment would detect a real difference, i.e. what sample size do you need? In clinical trials, the power is essential to see a treatment difference. A 90% power requirement means we want a 90% chance of detecting (value of variable measured) and require a sample size to be calculated (See Appendix 5). The power of a study is usually 80%, i.e. in 20% of cases we will miss the real difference and say there is no effect of the intervention in the experiment.

The power of a trial increases with increase in sample size. Estimating sample size is important because (i) if you use too large a sample you could waste time, money, and resources, e.g. doing a survey, (ii) if you use too small a sample you could get inaccurate results; there is less reliability on the sample data conclusions; you have to use less powerful statistical techniques for analysis, and it is difficult to infer conclusions about the population. Ideally you want a larger sample in order to make predictions about the population.

Repeating Measurements   It is essential to make sure that measurements are reliable (can be repeated – precision) and are valid (accurate). **Reliability** is the consistency or precision or repeatability of a measuring test. **Validity** is a measure of the accuracy of the test. A test is valid if it measures what it claims to measure. Consider the aim of using a dart to hit a target number of 20 on a dart board. Then our validity is how often we hit the number 20. The more times we hit 20, the more accurate the result. Our precision would also be high because we are repeatedly hitting the target. However, if we hit another number like 1 a high number of times, then our accuracy would be low but our precision would be high. The worst scenario is a low precision and a low accuracy (dart hits are all over the dart board).

So regular calibration (checking what is being measured with a reference or known values) and repeat measurements are essential.

In sampling data, how many replicates are used needs to be considered. **Replicates** are repeat measurements. Typically common is to do three, e.g. three samples of the same or three repeats of the same measurement. The analysis would then take the highest, the median, or the average of the replicates for further analysis. For example, in assays, measuring the concentrations or absorbances three times. In lung function tests, it is common to do three repetitions of the blowing manoeuvres.

Another factor to consider in repeating measurements is **order effects**. For example, if the experiment involves a physical activity, fatigue may occur, and so adequate rest needs to be included in the protocol. Increasing familiarity with an experiment or **learning effect** may also affect learning outcome, occur, and so **randomization** of the task needs to be considered. These should be discussed in choosing a study design. Listed below are some familiar designs reported in publications.

Common Examples of Study Design

1. **Repeated measures design**: each subject performs in both the control and experimental condition which could be more than one (e.g. three different treatments or conditions). For example, to see the effect of three different drugs in treating blood pressure, each subject receives a drug, and the effect on blood pressure is measured after 1 week. So, placebo (looks like the drug but does not have the active ingredient, e.g. sugar substitute) in one week, drugs A, B, and C in subsequent weeks. So, all subjects have received the same drugs. You could just have one drug, so the design would be paired, no treatment (no drug) or after treatment (receives drug). This is a strong design as the subject is acting as their own control and ruling out inter-subject variation.

2. **Independent subjects design**: some subjects perform in condition A and others in condition B. Subjects must be allocated randomly to each group. For example, two separate (unrelated or independent) groups of patients take drug A for a disease condition. Or two independent groups, one group taking drug A and the other taking drug B for a condition. You want to know which group shows a bigger response to the drug. The design is prone to within-subject and inter-subject variation.

3. **Matched pairs design**: from the results of a pre-test, the subjects are sorted into matched pairs (pairs of equal abilities on the task to be measured). One person from each pair performs in the experimental condition and one in the control. Suppose you had a group of patients with different levels of severity (e.g. difficulty in breathing). You would measure their lung function and then allocate them to groups based on severity (mild, moderate, and severe). Then each group would receive the same treatment or drug. This is a strong design due to matching the prior condition of the subjects.

4. **Cross-over design**: subjects are allocated randomly to either group A or group B. Group A does test 1 and group B does test 2. Then they cross over, Group B does test 1 and group A does test 2. If you had a group of subjects all with a similar condition, you would just randomly (e.g. assign a number to each subject) split them into two groups A and B, if you want to see the effect of two drugs D1 and D2. Then group A would be given D1 and group B would be given D2. They would then be measured to see the effect of the drug. Then group A would be given the other drug (D2) and group B would be given D1, and you would repeat the measurement. This is a strong design.

5. **Single blind design**: subjects are not aware whether they received the treatment or the placebo. This is common in clinical trials.

6. **Double blind design**: neither the subjects nor the researchers are aware who has taken the intervention (e.g. drug) and who has taken placebo, until after the experiment is completed. This is an extremely strong design and is considered the gold standard in clinical trials.

Carrying Out the Experiment

The above designs are incorporated into studies which vary in duration, size, and type.

Types of Studies A study conducted over a short time period with limited data is called a pilot study. The preliminary findings of this often lead to a longer study. Commonly, studies can be split into cross-sectional or longitudinal studies. **Cross-sectional studies** are studies in which subject data is collected once or more but in a short time period. **Longitudinal studies** are those in which subject data is collected over a long time period (months to years, e.g. epidemiological studies). Observation studies (with no intervention), involve data being collected over time to see how factors affecting disease vary. **Prospective studies** (forward looking) observe groups over time. **Retrospective studies** (backward looking) look back at groups who have been exposed to a condition. **Clinical trials** or experimental trials are studies where groups receive an intervention (e.g. therapy, test, or procedure) and they are compared to groups who did not receive the intervention.

In addition to studies collecting new data, studies are also published from use of existing data from published articles or analysis of accumulated data, e.g. hospital databases of patient data. Two examples of these are **systematic reviews** and **meta-analysis**. These studies are more common in clinical fields to review treatments and techniques. However, final year undergraduate projects are increasingly using these types of studies.

Systematic reviews identify, select, and critically appraise a specific aim or clearly defined question based on clear inclusion and exclusion criteria. It attempts to find all available information available and then to clearly state reasons for including and excluding studies. It then assesses the quality and bias of included studies and provides recommendations and suggestions for addressing any knowledge gaps in the area. For example, to review the situation about the current Corona virus, a systematic review was conducted by Park *et al.* (2020) called 'A Systematic Review of COVID-19 Epidemiology Based on Current Evidence'. For more information on conducting a systematic review please see the article by Wright *et al.* (2007).

Meta-analysis is a statistical technique to combine the findings of selected studies (based on inclusion and exclusion criteria, contains quantitative data) to critically answer a clearly defined aim or question. It uses statistical methods to evaluate, synthesize and summarize the study findings objectively. An example of a meta-analysis study can be seen in the paper by Bjordal *et al.* (2004). It can be done independently or as part of a systematic review. Examples of the types of plots (Forest and Funnel) produced in meta-analysis are shown in chapter 3.

After the Experiment

After collecting sample data which has been stored on computer software files and memory sticks, in laboratory notebooks or printed out, the data would then be displayed in tables and graphs.

Display of Data This is explored to look for any patterns or trends. These include seeing if the data are close together or spread out, and whether there is an increase, a decrease, or no change. However, these would be difficult to see if you had a large amount of data. To make this easier, data is displayed in tables and different types of graphs (see Chapter 2). The tables and graphs can display both the collected (raw) data and the calculated statistical data (which are also called summary statistics or descriptive statistics).

Summary Statistics   The summary statistics describe the data using statistical terms in two ways. One is the **central tendency** (middle), for example, using the word 'average' or 'mean'. The average will replace the raw data with one value. The second way is to describe the data in terms of how **spread out** it is, for example, using the word 'range' to describe the lowest (minimum) and highest (maximum) values. In this chapter we will explain mean and range, and also consider other terms to describe central tendency and spread of data in a sample taken from the population.

Let us look at some raw and statistical summary data to illustrate some of the terms described in this chapter (Table 1.1).

As you can see, the data is organized into three areas: the **variables**, the individual or **raw data**, and the **descriptive statistics**. The columns show the variables measured with their units. The rows show the individual data. The descriptive statistics in the last four rows show the number of subjects (**N**), the mean and the terms used to describe variation in the data, standard deviation (**±SD**) and the variation of the mean (**±SEM**) which show the error of the mean. The next section will describe and explain these descriptive statistics including the symbols used (see Appendix 2 & 3 for a list of common statistical terms & symbols) and show examples of how to calculate them.

> *"He who loves practice without theory is like the sailor who boards ship without a rudder and compass and never knows where he may be cast."*
> – Leonardo da Vinci (1452–1519) – artist, engineer

Descriptive Statistics

We have explained above that descriptive statistics summarize raw data. We will now describe more terms used to summarize data, i.e. the size of a sample, the shape of distribution (e.g. normal or bell shaped), central tendency (e.g. mean, mode, median) and the variability of the sample data (e.g. standard deviation, variance, range)

Sample Size

This is the total number of observations or data, the common symbol used is N. This is very important, particularly if it is small because: (i) if N is small it is difficult to make conclusions about the population, (ii) it is difficult to use more powerful statistical tests such as parametric tests, (iii) it is difficult to make conclusions of clinical importance, (iv) it is difficult to show reproducibility or precision, (v) when high percentages are mentioned, the sample size could be very small (e.g. in surveys, advertising, polling). If N is large (typically > 30), then the sample distribution (see Chapter 3) will approximate more to the population distribution (sample mean and variance similar to population mean and variance).

TABLE 1.1 Subject details and changes in heart rate and minute ventilation at rest and exercise. HR = heart rate; VE = minute ventilation; N = sample size; VE = minute ventilation; SD = standard deviation; SEM = standard error of the mean

SUBJECT	GENDER	AGE Yrs	WEIGHT Kg	HEIGHT Cm	REST HR (b/min)	REST VE (l/min)	EXERCISE HR (b/min)	EXERCISE VE (l/min)
1	M	21	58	171	113	14.4	131	33.8
2	M	24	85	182	87	14.5	95	28.3
3	F	23	63	160	81	16.4	137	23.4
4	M	26	73	174	115	24.2	114	24.2
5	M	20	77	178	70	24.8	84	26.7
6	M	20	66	175	61	12.6	91	19.3
7	F	20	58	161	82	15.0	100	26.0
8	F	20	60	180	110	20.3	142	22.3
N		8	8	8	8	8	8	8
MEAN		21.8	67.5	1726	89.8	17.8	111.7	25.5
±SD		23	9.9	8.2	20.6	4.7	22.6	4.4
±SEM		0.8	3.5	2.9	7.3	1.7	8.0	1.5

Annotations:

- Rows contain the raw data
- Conditions or interventions- independent variables, rest and exercise. HR = heart rate
- Measured variables- dependent variables, HR, VE
- Variables of personal characteristics of subjects, gender, age, weight, height
- Columns contain the variables
- Table number and title and legend or key to describe the symbols used placed on top of table
- These 4 rows contain the descriptive stats (N, mean, SD, SEM.
- Size of sample.
- Average of the sample data (central tendency)
- Standard error of the mean- describes the accuracy of finding the mean
- Standard deviation- describes variability of the sample data (measure of spread of the data)

Measures of Central Tendency

Mean   Is the arithmetic average of all the values in a sample of data, i.e. the sum of all the data divided by the number of data. The symbol used is $\bar{X}$ (x bar). If we knew the mean of the data from the total population, then the symbol used would be μ (mu).

Mean $(\bar{X})$ = sum of data/number of data = $\Sigma x/N$

where x = data value; Σx = sum of data; N = total number of data.

It is a measure of the central tendency (middle or centre) of set of data. It is markedly affected by very high or low values which are called outliers. It doesn't give information about the spread of the data. There are errors in calculating the mean as above if the scale of the measurements is not linear (e.g. pH is a log scale), if you are using ratios or percentages, finding the overall mean of sample means if the sample sizes are different. For example, mean blood pressure (pressure exerted in arterial blood vessels by the heart) is often quoted as 120/80, where the top figure is the systolic pressure (highest pressure generated by the heart) and the bottom figure is diastolic pressure (resting pressure of the heart).

Importance of the mean

- The most common and frequently used term to describe the central or middle view of data is the mean. The median and mode are not used as frequently.
- In inferential tests (hypothesis tests), differences in the mean between two or more groups are tested using probability.
- Experiments report the accuracy of the sample mean as an estimate of the population mean using standard errors and confidence intervals.

The symbol Σ is called sigma. It is the sum or total from adding several items of data. Suppose we have three data values called x_1, x_2, x_3, then the sum would be:
$\Sigma = x_1 + x_2 + x_3$

Franklin D. Roosevelt

An American president who died in 1945 aged 63 years from cerebral haemorrhage (stroke) had a blood pressure of 300/190, an extreme case of hypertension!

EXAMPLE 1.1 | Calculation of the mean

Students were asked to hold their breath as long as possible after filling their lungs with air to maximum. The breath hold times in seconds measured with a stopwatch were:

55, 60, 50, 67, 71, 78, 75, 80, 84, 52, 65

Step 1: Count the number of sample data: here $N = 11$
Step 2: Find the sum of the sample data: here $\Sigma x = 737$
Step 3: Divide the sum of the data by the sample size

Thus, mean $(\bar{x})$ = sum of data/number of data = $\Sigma x/N$
or mean = 737/11 = 67 s

Median   This is the central or middle value of a group of data, after the data is ordered (low to high). Unlike the mean it is not affected by extreme values (very low or very high values), however, it doesn't give the spread of the data. If there is an even number of data, then there will be two middle numbers, in which case the average of the two numbers will give the median.

EXAMPLE 1.2 | Calculation of the median for an odd sample

For the above breath data: 55, 60, 50, 67, 71, 78, 75, 80, 84, 52, 65

Step 1: First put the data in order of increasing size
      50, 52, 55, 60, 65, 67, 71, 75, 78, 80, 84

Step 2: Find the middle number: in this case it is 67 s (with five numbers to the left of 67 and five numbers to the right of 67).

In an odd sample, the middle value can be found easily.

EXAMPLE 1.3 | Calculation of the Median for an even sample

If we added an extra student's breath hold time (e.g. 65 s) to the above data, we will now have an even sample of data:

55, 60, 50, 67, 71, 78, 75, 80, 84, 52, 65, 65

Step 1: Put sample data in order
      50, 52, 55, 60, 65, 65, 67, 71, 75, 78, 80, 84

Step 2: In an even sample there will be two middle values, Identify the two middle numbers, i.e. 65 and 67

Step 3: Calculate the median by taking the average of the two middle numbers, i.e. median = (65 + 67)/2 = 66 s.

Mode   The mode is the value that appears most frequently (largest frequency). In a sample of data, the number of times a number occurs is counted.

EXAMPLE 1.4 | Calculation of the Mode

Volunteers in a research study had their weight in kg measured as shown below:

50, 50, 52, 55, 60, 65, 65, 65, 67, 71, 75, 78, 80, 84

EXAMPLE 1.4 *(continued)*

Step 1: Examine the data and count the number of times a number appears in the sample data. For the above data, we can see that the number 50 occurs twice, whilst the number 65 occurs three times, the rest of the numbers appear once.

Step 2: Therefore

The mode = the value which appears most frequently is = 65 kg.

Standard Error of the Mean (SEM) The mean of a sample is usually stated with a number called the standard error of the mean (SEM), which is an estimate of the precision of estimating the population mean. It is a measure of the accuracy of the mean. It would be written as mean ± SEM, where the ± SEM defines the range, interval, or band where the mean could be.

For example, if the mean red blood cell count from eight healthy subjects was $5.8 \pm$ SEM 0.8 mill μL^{-1}.
The lower limit would be $5.8 - 0.8 = 5$ mill μL^{-1}
The upper limit would be $5.8 + 0.8 = 6.6$ mill μL^{-1}

Thus, the mean could be between 5 mill μL^{-1} to 6.6 mill μL^{-1} for this sample. You can compare your mean red blood cell count to published population means for red blood cell counts to see if it was normal or abnormal.

To understand SEM, consider the measurement of the weights of students in one classroom. We can calculate the mean for this classroom. This mean value will be in a range with an upper and lower limit just like the red blood cell count above. We can take a second sample by repeating the weights of students in another classroom and again we will have a mean and a range where the mean might be defined by an upper limit and a lower limit. This range where the mean could be found is called the standard error of the mean for that sample. If we now do this for all the classrooms in the school, we will have an overall mean. This overall mean is the population mean (the population would be all the classes in the school). So having more samples and larger samples would give us a mean which more accurately represents the population mean.

If the SEM range is small, then there is more accuracy in determining the mean. A smaller range is favoured if the sample size is large and there is a small variation of data (small standard deviation or variance). Another

---

SEM

- Is a measure of the precision or accuracy of the sample mean as an estimate of the population mean.
- Is equal to the standard deviation/square root of sample size.
- Is useful for calculating the confidence interval
- Decreases as sample size increases.
- If you repeat an experiment and each time calculate the sample mean, then the SD of the sample means is called the SEM.

term which is used to give an estimate of finding the mean is the confidence interval (see below). The standard deviation and variance are measures of the spread of data (see below). The standard error of the mean is equal to the standard deviation divided by the square root of the sample size.

$$SEM = SD/\sqrt{N}$$

EXAMPLE 1.5 | Calculation of the standard error of the mean (SEM)

Consider the breath hold data from Example 1.1.

55, 60, 50, 67, 71, 78, 75, 80, 84, 52, 65

Step 1: Calculate the standard deviation (SD) of the sample data
Step 2: Find the square root of N
Step 3: Divide the SD by the square root of N

$$SEM = 11.704/\sqrt{11} = 3.53 \text{ s}$$

Step 4: Thus the ± SEM is = ± 3.53 s

Step 5: Since the mean is 67 s, then the mean breath hold ± SEM = 67 ± 3.53 s

The mean is the most common measure of central location or central tendency. However, as we have mentioned it is affected by large or small values and so the median avoids this, but it doesn't show the spread of the data. You will need to see which best describes your data, by exploring your data by graphical methods (see Chapter 2).

Variation of Data

The variation of the data (also known as dispersion or spread) can be described by the range, standard deviation, variance, coefficient of variation, quartiles, interquartile range, and percentiles. These will be described below.

Range   This is a measure of the spread of the data, from the smallest to the largest size of your sample data. It is calculated by the largest value subtracting the smallest value. The disadvantage of the range is that it doesn't show the scatter of the data and extreme values affect it.

In biosciences, a special form of range called the **reference range** is very important particularly in disease diagnosis and to see whether you are in the normal range. These reference ranges are obtained from collating data from large studies. Consider the reference range for blood pressure in normal and hypertension (sustained and elevated blood pressure) conditions. The World Health Organization (WHO) define the following reference ranges for blood pressure:

EXAMPLE 1.6 | Calculation of the Range

For the sample data of age (years) of subjects:

18, 27, 45, 23, 27, 30

Step 1: Examine the data and identify the largest and smallest values; in this case it is
45 and 18 respectively
Step 2: Calculate the range

Range = highest value – lowest = 45 – 18 = 27 years.

115/75 to 120/80 mmHg is normal
120/80 to 139/89 mmHg is pre-hypertension
140/90 to 159/99 mmHg is stage 1 hypertension
>160/ > 100 mmHg is stage 2 hypertension

Regular measurements of blood pressure can then
be used to monitor and assess the effect of the
interventions of anti-hypertensive drugs or lifestyle
changes (e.g. diet, exercise) on the blood pressure.

In disease diagnosis, body fluids (e.g. urine,
saliva, cerebrospinal fluid) are sampled. One of the
most common body fluids which is regularly sampled is blood. A blood sample will
have many reference ranges for a wide number of variables (Figure 1.2).

> *Blood Glucose (fasting) levels
> (from the National Institute for
> Clinical Excellence)*
>
> Normal: 4–5.6 mmol L^{-1}
> (72–100 mg/100 mL blood)
> Pre-diabetic: 5.6–6.9 mmol L^{-1}
> (100–125 mg/100 mL
> Diabetic: > 7 mmol L^{-1}
> (126 mg/100 mL)

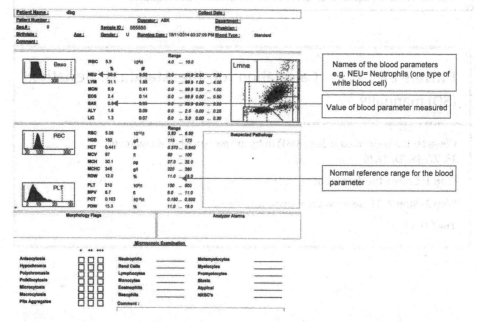

FIGURE 1.2   Blood parameters and reference ranges (from one person) using Pentra 60
Blood Analyser.

SD

- Is a measure of variability of sample data.
- It is an estimate of the variability of the population from which the sample is taken.
- SD^2 = variance.
- In a normal distribution, 95% of data will be within ± 2 SD.

Note: if the population is sampled, then the $(N-1)$ is replaced by N in the formula for SD and the symbol used for population standard deviation is σ (sigma)

Standard Deviation (SD)   This is a measure of the distribution of data around the mean; i.e. how far away from the mean an individual value lies. If the data is normally distributed, then SD tells us what proportion of the scores falls within certain limits: e.g. 68% of scores lie within ± 1 SD of the mean; 95% between ± 2 SD of the mean, and 99.7% lie within ±3 SD.

The larger the SD, the larger the range of values (variation) in the data.

The SD can be calculated for a sample dataset using the formula below.

SD = Square root of (sum of squares/ degrees of freedom)
$$= \sqrt{[(\Sigma x_i - \overline{x}) / N - 1)]}.$$

Where, $\overline{x} = mean$; X_i = each data value; $\Sigma(x_i - \overline{x})^2$ = sum of squares; N = sample size; $N-1$ = degrees of freedom

---

Sum of squares

- Suppose we have three data values called $X1, X2, X3$ and the mean of these three values was $\overline{x}$.
- The difference between each data value and the mean would be $(X1 - \overline{x})$, $(X2 - \overline{x})$, $(X3 - \overline{x})$.
- The square of each difference would be $(X1 - \overline{x})^2$, $(X2 - \overline{x})^2$, $(X3 - \overline{x})^2$.
- The sum of these squared differences would be the sum of squares.

EXAMPLE 1.7 | Calculation of the standard deviation (SD) manually

Consider the body mass index (BMI) in kg m^{-2} measured in six women:
18, 27, 45, 23, 27, 30

Step 1: Collate the data (Table 1.2).

Step 2–Step 7: These steps are shown in Table 1.2.

The SD = 9.16

TABLE 1.2 Manual calculation of the standard deviation (SD) for values (x)

	x	$x_i - \bar{x}$	$(x_i - \bar{x})^2$
	18	-10.33	106.71
	27	-1.33	1.77
	45	16.67	277.89
	23	-5.33	28.41
	27	-1.33	1.77
	30	1.67	2.79
Mean	$\bar{x} = 28.33$		
Sum of squares			$\sum (x_i - \bar{x})^2$ 419.34
SD = Square root of (sum of squares/degrees of freedom)			$(\sum(x_i - \bar{x})^2)/(N-1) =$ $\sqrt{(419.34/5)} =$ $\sqrt{83.87} = 9.16$

Step 2: Find the mean of your data

Step 3: Subtract the mean from each value i.e. $x_i - \bar{x}$

Step 4: Square the answer in step 3

Step 5: Add the answers of step 3 (i.e. sum of squares)

Step 6: Divide the sum of squares by the degrees of freedom

Step 7: Take the square root of the answer for step 6

Variance   This is an estimate of variability. It measures how far every data is from the mean and from each other. Thus, a small variance indicates that the data is close to the mean and to other values. It is very closely related to standard deviation, since the square of the standard deviation is equal to variance, i.e. **SD² = variance**. It is easier to work with mathematically, since SD has positive and negative values.

Variance = sum of squares/degrees of freedom

$$= (\sum(x_i - \bar{x})^2/(N-1)$$

Where, $\bar{x} = mean$, N-1 = degrees of freedom, x_i = each value of sample, $(x_i - \bar{x})^2$ = sum of squares

---

EXAMPLE 1.8 | Calculation of the variance manually

Consider the BMI data from Example 1.7.
18, 27, 45, 23, 27, 30

Step 1: Tabulate the data (Table 1.3) and find the mean of the data
Step 2: Subtract the mean from each value,, i.e. $x_i - \bar{x}$
Step 3: Square the answer in step 2
Step 4: Add the answers of step 3 (i.e. sum of squares)
Step 5: Dividing the sum of squares by the degrees of freedom gives the variance

Thus, the variance is 83.87. If we take the square root of this, we will obtain the SD, which is 9.16.

TABLE 1.3 Manual calculation of variance for data (x)

x	$x_i - \bar{x}$	$(x_i - \bar{x})^2$
18	-10.33	106.71
27	-1.33	1.77
45	16.67	277.89
23	-5.33	28.41
27	-1.33	1.77
30	1.67	2.79
Mean	$\bar{x} = 28.33$	
Sum of squares	$\left(\sum(x_i - \bar{x})^2 = 419.34\right)$	
Variance (sum of squares/degrees of freedom)	$\left(\sum(x_i - \bar{x})^2\right)/(N-1)$ $=419.34/5=83.87$	

Coefficient of Variation (CV%)   The coefficient of variation (CV) is a measure of the variation of data. It is the standard deviation divided by the mean and expressed as a percentage. The higher the CV, the more variable the data.

$$\text{CV (\%)} = (\text{SD/mean}) \times 100$$

Variance

- Is a measure of variability of sample data.
- Variance = square of the standard deviation (SD^2).
- Equal or unequal variance between two groups has to be tested before an independent t-test.
- Variance is compared between multiple groups in parametric tests such as ANOVA.

EXAMPLE 1.9 | Calculation of the Coefficient of variation (CV)

Consider the BMI data below:
18, 27, 45, 23, 27, 30

Step 1: Calculate the mean of the data, i.e. mean = 28.33
Step 2: Calculate the standard deviation of the data, i.e. SD = 9.16
Step 3: Divide the standard deviation by the mean and convert to a percentage by multiplying by 100, i.e. CV = (SD/Mean) x 100 = (9.16/28.33) x 100 = 32%

Quartiles   The spread of sample data can also be described by splitting the data into four quartiles after putting them in order. The quartiles are split between the minimum value and the maximum value. Each quartile represents 25% of the data. The **first quartile (Q1)** describes 25% of the data below and 75% above it. The **second quartile (Q2)** represents 50% of the data below and 50% of the data above it. And the **third quartile** represents 75% of the data below it and 25% of the data above it. The **fourth quartile** has all the data below it. The **interquartile range (Q3–Q1)** represents the middle 50% of the data. These quartiles are displayed graphically in a box and whisker plot (see Chapter 2) and below (Figure 1.3). The box shows the middle part of the data. Quartiles are useful to see if data is skewed either to the lower or to the higher values, so it is a measure of variability.

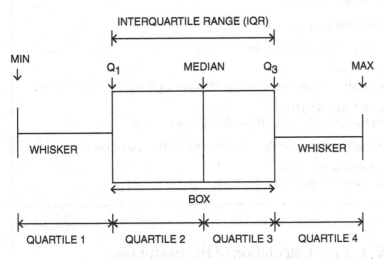

FIGURE 1.3   Sample data split into quartiles on a box and whisker plot.

If we measured the cholesterol levels of a group of subjects and displayed the results as quartiles in a box and whisker plot, we would know the following information: (i) what the lowest (minimum) and highest (maximum) cholesterol for the group is; (ii) the middle 50% of the group's cholesterol (from the interquartile range); the middle value (median) cholesterol for the group. For any individual we would know whether they were in the high cholesterol, low cholesterol, or middle range of values and where the value lies in relation to others in the group.

Percentiles   Sample data can also be described by percentiles which are very similar to quartiles. Data which has been put in order are divided into 100ths or percentages. A percentile describes a score which describes what percentage of the other values are below it. For example, if your score is 68 and this is ranked as the 75th percentile, then 75% of the data values in the sample are below 68. Percentiles can be calculated using the formula: ***Percentile = (number of values below score)×(total number of values)/ 100***

The range and the interquartile range indicate overall variation in a dataset, but they don't show the detailed spread of the data. Standard deviation and variance show this detail. Variance is a more convenient way of looking at spread of data as it doesn't involve the negative numbers of standard deviation. Plotting data graphically (see Chapter 2) for example box and whisker plots or frequency distributions will not only show the spread of data but also the central location of data.

EXAMPLE 1.10 | Calculation of quartiles

Ten students produced a blood smear glass slide. The slides were assessed for their quality and the following scores (out of 100) were given. Find the first, second, third quartiles and the interquartile range.

55, 30, 48, 51, 37, 66, 86, 73, 68, 75

Step 1: Put the numbers in order

30, 37, 48, 51, 55, 66, 68, 73, 75, 86

Step 2: Find the median
The two middle numbers are 55 and 66. Thus the median = (55 + 66)/2 = 60.5

Step 3: Find the first quartile (Q1)
From the numbers below 60.5, the middle number is = 48

Step 4: Find the middle number for the values above 60.5, the middle number = 73

Step 5: Find the interquartile range
The interquartile range = Q3-Q1 = 73–48 = 25

EXAMPLE 1.11 | Calculation of the percentile

In a reaction time test on a computer to the following scores (out of 100) were given. Calculate the percentile of the person who scored 73.

55, 30, 48, 51, 37, 66, 86, 73, 68, 75

Step 1: Put the scores in order
30, 37, 48, 51, 55, 66, 68, 73, 75, 86

Step 2: Count the number of values below the score of 73.
This is 7.

Step 3: Count the total number of scores.
This is 10.

Step 4: Calculate the percentile
Percentile = (number of values below the score of 73) x (total number of scores)/100)
Or = 7/ (10 x100)
= (7 x 10)/100
= 0.7
Or 70%.
This means that 70% of the scores were below 73.

Confidence Interval

To understand the concept of confidence interval better, the reader should read about probability (frequency) distributions like the normal distribution (t and Z distributions) in Chapter 2 and look at Chapter 3 to see how it relates to probability.

If studies were repeated on different random groups from a population, a range of results would be obtained (each random group will have different means and standard deviations). The confidence interval (CI) represents the intervals or range of values in which the mean occurs, i.e. a measure of reliability of the mean occurring. The CI can also be considered as a measure of the uncertainty in finding the mean.

> **Confidence Interval**
>
> - Is a measure of the certainty of finding the mean at different confidence levels.
> - The most common CI is the 95%.
> - For a large sample, 95% CI = mean ± 1.96 SEM.
> - For small samples, 95% CI = mean ± t_{value} SEM.
> - A 95% CI implies that if you did an experiment 100 times, in 95 experiments you will include the mean.
> - CI takes into account sample size, standard error and probability.
> - CI decrease with increase in sample size as we obtain a better estimate of the population mean.
> - Both CI and SEM describe the error of estimating the population mean, however the CI shows the error based on different confidence levels.

The CI is expressed by two parts:

i. **A range or interval**: an upper estimate and lower estimate, e.g. the blood pressure measured from a sample of data could have a CI between 115 and 125 mmHg.

ii. **Level of the confidence interval:** as a percentage (e.g. 99%, 95%, 90%). A 95% CI states that we have a 95% chance of finding the true population mean within the interval.

If we want a higher CI to find the mean, then the probability or reliability of finding the mean decreases. For example, a 99% CI is wider than a 95% CI which is wider than a 90% CI. But the probability of finding the mean is more difficult the wider the confidence interval as you are increasing the margin of error. So, the best compromise and most widely used confidence interval is the 95% CI. The narrower the confidence interval, the more accurately we can predict the true mean value.

The CI can be calculated for means, medians, proportions, correlations, and regression coefficients. It is affected by the sample size, standard deviation (SD), and the level of confidence. There are slightly different formulas for the CI depending on the size of the sample and whether the population standard deviation is known.

Formula 1. If the sample size is less than 30 and the population SD is unknown then use:

CI= mean ± t_{value} x SEM
Or,
CI= mean ± t_{value} x SD/$\sqrt{N}$

where t_{value} = value corresponding to $p = 0.05$ and degrees of freedom (N-1).
SD = sample standard deviation
Mean = sample mean
Note: SD/$\sqrt{N}$ is also the standard error (SEM);
t_{value} x SD/$\sqrt{N}$ is also called the margin of error (ME)

Sample size affects SEM and the width of the confidence interval. The smaller the sample the less accurate is the standard error and the wider the confidence interval width, i.e. there is less likelihood of finding the true mean. So, a sample size of 100 will have a wider CI compared to a sample size of 1000. If zero is within the CI, this suggests a non-significant result; if zero is outside the CI, this suggests significance.

Formula 2. If the sample size is greater than 30, and we know the population SD, then use:

$$CI = mean \pm Z\ SEM$$

Where mean = sample mean,
SEM = standard error (or SD/$\sqrt{N}$);
    Z = confidence level value

---

t_{value}

- Are standardized values calculated from sample data which are used in hypothesis tests.
- A t_{value} is calculated by dividing the difference between the means of two samples by the standard error.
- Are used in hypothesis tests to show whether differences in means between two samples occurred by chance.
- The t_{values} form a probability distribution very similar to the normal distribution.
- Every t_{value} is associated with a P value and degree of freedom.
- P value is a number (between 0 and 1 or 0 and 100%) which states the probability of an event happening. A P of 5% (=0.05) means there is a 1 in 20 chance of an event happening.
- Degree of freedom is related to sample size, it is your sample size minus 1. It is measure of the number of values in a data sample that have the freedom to vary.

$$CI = mean \pm t_{value} \times SD/\sqrt{N}$$

Z value

- Z values (or Z scores) are standardized values obtained from sample data values which come from a population with a normal distribution, with known population mean and standard deviation.
- Z = (sample data value − population mean)/population standard deviation.
- Z values describe the variation of sample values in SD from the mean.
- Z values form a standard normal distribution (frequency of Z against SD) with mean of zero.
- Z values are negative below the mean and positive above the mean.
- The importance of Z values are (i) they allow us to find the probability of a sample data occurring in a normal distribution, and (ii) compare two sample data values from two different normal distributions.
- Advantage of Z scores is that they show how an individual compares with other people. For example your marks for a biochemistry and microbiology module test could be compared more accurately with other people if the marks were converted to Z scores, i.e. we are all using the same scale.

If we know the mean and standard deviation of a group of sample data, we can convert every data point in the sample to a standard score or Z score. Z is known as a standard score or Z score, has a distribution, and is a measure of the standard deviation above and below the population mean. It is used to compare sample results to the normal population. Z can be defined by the following formula.

Z = (observed value – sample mean)/standard deviation of sample.
Or,
$Z = (X - \bar{x})/SD$

Note if the population mean or standard deviation is known, then these would be used in the formula. We could replace Z score with a t score from the t distribution, to calculate the confidence interval. The sample size affects t, but when the sample size is > 30 then t is quite close to the value of Z, we can then use, $Z = 1.96$, as the critical value for a 95% confidence interval.

EXAMPLE 1.12 | Calculation of the confidence interval from sample data

Consider the breath hold times in seconds from example 1.1.
55, 60, 50, 67, 71, 78, 75, 80, 84, 52, 65

Step 1: Calculate the standard deviation: SD = 11.704 s
Step 2: Calculate the mean: 67 s
Step 3: Calculate the standard error of the mean (SEM): here SEM = 3.529 s
Step 4: Note the sample size and degree of freedom, i.e,. N = 11; degree of freedom $(N-1)$ = 10
Step 5: Using the tables for t values (see Appendix 8) and the degree of freedom of 10, find the t value, i.e. 2.228
Step 6: Calculate the margin of error (ME)
    Where, ME = (t value for $n–1$ degrees of freedom x SD)/square root of N
    Or ME = t value for $n–1$ degrees of freedom x SEM
    Or ME = 2.228 x 3.529 = 7.86

Step 7: Calculate the confidence interval
    CI = mean ± ME
    CI = 67 ± ((2.228 x 11.704)/ $\sqrt{N}$) = 67 ±7.86 = 59.14 to 74.86

EXAMPLE 1.13 | Calculation of the confidence interval with known mean and SD

Forty students had their systolic blood pressure measured and the mean was 123 mmHg with a SD of 8 mmHg.
a) Find the 95% confidence interval

EXAMPLE 1.13 *(continued)*

---

b) Find the 99% confidence interval

Step 1: The formula for the 95% confidence interval is shown below, state the values for the parts of the formula

Or confidence interval is between mean + t (SD/$\sqrt{N}$) and mean − t (SD/$\sqrt{N}$)
SD = 8, mean = 123, N = 40, df = 40-1 = 39, t = 2.02 (from table of critical values df = 39, and P = 0.05), SEM = (SD/$\sqrt{N}$) = 8/$\sqrt{40}$ = 1.24

Step 2: Put values into formula
123 + 2.02 (8/$\sqrt{40}$) and 123−2.02 (8/$\sqrt{40}$)

Or 95% confidence interval is 120.4 to 125.6 mmHg

Step 3: For the 99% confidence interval, substitute a new t value of 2.70 (from df of 39 and P = 0.01 and critical table)
Thus, confidence interval is

123 ± 2.70(8/$\sqrt{40}$)

Or 99% confidence interval is 119.6 to 126.4 mmHg.

CI = mean ± 1.96 SEM This gives the values between which 95% confidence of finding the mean, i.e. we can be 95% certain that the true mean value lies within ± 2 standard deviations.

Interpretation: in theory, our population mean would be between 120.4 mmHg and 125.6 mmHg. However, this is not correct, since one sample is not representative of the population. You would have to take many samples and work out CI for each sample, and then from these estimated CI you could more accurately predict the population mean. We can see that the 99% CI is wider than the 95% CI, which means that the uncertainty in finding the population mean is greater in the 99% than in the 95% CI.

Degrees of Freedom

The degrees of freedom are a measure of the ability (or 'freedom') of values or variables to vary.

Suppose you have a bag containing five different coloured balls, where the variable is the colour of the ball. If you take out one of the balls from the bag, then you have decreased your degree of freedom by one to choose from the five colours. If you take out another ball you have decreased your degree of freedom even further, and so on.

Suppose we have N observations in a sample, then each is free to have any value, but if you calculate the sample mean, then you restrict the value of the test measurement, i.e. your degree of freedom is restricted. Hence the degree of freedom mathematically $= N-1$.

> **"... the actual and physical conduct of an experiment must govern the statistical procedure of its interpretation."**
> *Ronald Aylmer Fisher (1890–1962)- British mathematician, Biologist*

Summary

- Data can be obtained from population samples or total populations.
- Data types: quantitative (continuous, discrete); qualitative (ordinal, nominal).
- Data samples are described by descriptive statistics as measures of central location or central tendency (mean, mode, median) and the spread (variation) of the data (standard deviation, variance, quartiles, interquartile range, percentiles).
- Sample data is used to make predictions about the population data.
- Sample data are used to produce probability (frequency) distributions (e.g. normal, t, Z).
- Population data have a population mean and population standard deviation.
- Sample data have a sample mean and sample standard deviation.
- Standard error describes the error of the sample mean from the actual mean of the population and standard deviation is a measure of the variability of sample data around the mean.
- The accuracy of the mean is described by the confidence interval (usually the 95%) and standard error.
- The mean is a very important statistic as it describes the central tendency of data and is used in comparing differences between samples in hypothesis testing.
- The variation of the data is most commonly described by standard deviation and variance.
- The reference range is an important guide in defining normal and abnormal values, e.g. in diagnosis and treatment of disease, accuracy of instrumentation.
- Experiments need a clear aim, experimental design, a control, and adequate sample size.
- Data can be collected from different types of studies such as epidemiological, clinical trials, and experiments.

Sample Problems

Answers to all sample problems are found in Appendix 7.

Type of data

1) Describe the following data using the terms, quantitative, qualitative, discrete, continuous, ordinal, and nominal:
(i) Ethnicity of volunteers, (ii) number of red blood cells counted on a haemocytometer, (iii) Borg's perceived rate of exertion, (iv) metabolic rate measured from a wet spirometer, (v) size of Bowman's capsule in a kidney

Descriptive Statistics

2) The following weights in grams were obtained from male Wistar rats. Calculate the descriptive statistics (mean, median, mode, range, SD, SEM) for the following data:
200, 250, 400, 350, 520, 324, 568, 425, 300, 236, 185, 520, 250, 300, 350, 400, 300

Confidence Interval and Coefficient of Variation

3) Calculate the 95% confidence interval (CI) and the coefficient of variation for the measurements of a volume of 4000 μL^{-1} of red blood cell diluting fluid measured with a Gilson pipette (P5000) by 12 students.
4100, 3980, 3990, 4200, 3700, 4300, 4500, 4000, 3995, 4005

CHAPTER 2

Displaying and Exploring Sample Data Graphically

"The greatest value of a picture is when it forces us to notice what we never expected to see."

John Tukey (1915–2000) - American mathematician, statistician

Expected Learning Outcomes

- Present data in tables.
- Present data in graphs.
- Describe the importance of the normal distribution.
- Extract information from tables, graphs and normal distributions.
- Explain the purpose of error bars.

Data are displayed in tables and graphs. In most publications there is a combination of tables and graphs.

Presenting Data in Tables

Tables are useful for the initial record of the data values (raw values) and then further tables are produced from this raw data to show the descriptive statistics (such as the means, SD (standard deviation) and SEM (standard error of the mean)) which summarizes the central tendency and spread of the data.

....

Essential Statistics for Bioscientists, First Edition. Mohammed Meah.
© 2022 John Wiley & Sons Ltd. Published 2022 by John Wiley & Sons Ltd.

Tables are also useful because you can see the actual values, can show transformations of the data in other columns and can store large amounts of information. Raw data and mean data of marks obtained for various assessments in a module for seven students is given in Table 2.1.

TABLE 2.1 **Student assessment and module marks**
Dependent variables

Student	Exam	Lab Report	Critical Appraisal	Reflection	Presentation	Module Marks
	%	%	%	%	%	%
1	72.7	80	80	90	90.3	79
2	44.0	70	70	80	66.5	54
3	57.3	60	68	65	68.9	62
4	63.0	76	95	70	83.1	72
5	68.3	40	65	60	72.9	69
6	49.7	47	45	50	42.8	47
7	53.0	80	70	75	88.1	67
N	7	7	7	7	7	7
Mean	58.3	64.7	70.4	70.0	73.2	64.3
±SD	10.3	16.2	15.2	13.2	16.3	10.9
±SEM	3.9	6.1	5.7	5.0	6.2	4.1

Independent variables

Descriptive Statistics

Each table should have a table number and informative title above the table. There should be a brief explanatory legend to explain abbreviations and symbols used, and any relevant information about the experiment.

The table structure and style will vary, but typically, you show **dependent variables** data (groups, controls, variables) with their relevant units and **independent variables** (e.g. subjects, time). Note: if it is subjects, we need to anonymize by using subject number or initials, so that personal information cannot be identified by people not associated with the study. The data should normally be shown with one or two decimal places. At the end of the columns there would be **descriptive statistics** (N (size of sample), mean, SD (standard deviation) and SEM (standard error of the mean)). P values (dealing with significance of mean differences) are normally shown with asterisks and explained in the legend. A popular spreadsheet used to produce tables is an Excel spreadsheet.

Typically, in publications or posters it is commonly mean data that is shown in a table. Table 2.2 shows the mean changes in parameters which measure the variation of heart beats (heart rate variability) in 24 subjects while their body position was tilted to different angles and they performed handgrip exercise. The rows show the dependent variables and the columns show the independent variables.

> **"If I can't picture it, I can't understand it."**
> -Albert Einstein (1879–1955)
> - Physicist

TABLE 2.2   **Effect of stressors on heart rate variability parameters**

Independent Variables

Parameters	TT Control	IHG Control	TT 60	IHG+TT60	TT80	IHG+TT80
Heart Rate (bpm)	72.8±2.3	75.4±2.3	80.5±1.9	83.8±2.0	83.5±1.9	85.0±2.0
SDNN(ms)	133.3±27.2	130.6±26.6	96.0±19.6	83.9±17.1	90.4±18.4	91.54±18.6
SDSD(ms)	107.6±13.5	80.7±13.4	75.7±9.4	46.7±6.2	73.8±9.5	42.5±6.1
pNN50%	16.6±2.1	13.4±2.1	8.5±1.1	6.0±1.3	6.8±0.9	6.0±1.0
LF%	11.5±2.0	12.9±2.5	14.9±3.01	16.1±3.3	15.3±2.7	13.6±2.5
HF%	19.8±4.2	15.2±3.5	14.2±3.3	11.0±3.0	13.1±3.2	6.0±1.9
LF/HF ratio%	10.5±1.7	25.2±7.4	21.1±4.5	34.5±7.6	28.8±6.2	54±14.1

KEY: Mean (N=24±SEM) HRV during head up tilting (TT) and isometric hand grip exercise (IHG):TT60 & TT80=tilting at 60 and 80 degrees; IHG + TT60=80=tilting and handgrip At 60 and 80 degrees.

Dependent Variables

Presenting Data in Graphs

Displaying data in graphical form allows us to see the structure of the data. We can see if there have been any increases or decreases in the means, the spread of the data and if there are any outliers (extreme values), or if there are any trends, or if there are any correlations (links or associations) between variables. So graphically exploring raw data is recommended at the end of data collection. Ideally for publications, graphical presentation of data is the most popular choice.

General Features of Graphs

It is common to plot graphs with the **dependent variables on the vertical (y) axis** and the **independent variables on the horizontal (x) axis**. In Figure 2.1, absorbance is a ratio and has no units. The equation and R shows strength of the linear relationship between absorbance and concentration (see Chapter 4).

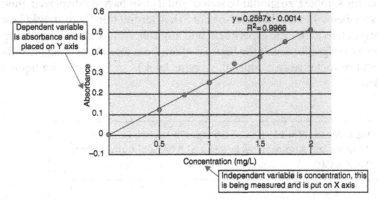

FIGURE 2.1   Light absorbance against potassium dichromate concentration.

The independent variable is the factor that is controlled or manipulated by the experimenter (e.g. time, concentration, treatment, intervention). The dependent variable depends on the independent variable and is the one being measured (gives the results of the experiment e.g. response, absorbance, temperature).

Some graphs will have two y axes to represent two separate variables. In Figure 2.2 below, one y axis represents blood pressure and the other represents heart rate.

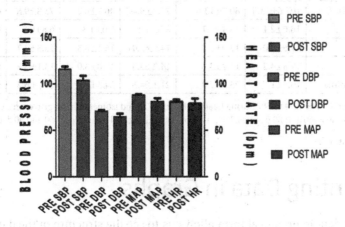

FIGURE 2.2   Mean (N = 10) ± SEM blood pressure and heart rate pre and post slow breathing training.

Size of graph   The graph size should generally be large, making full use of the axes so that data points can be seen clearly (e.g. 1/4 to 1/3 of a page) otherwise it is difficult to read.

Title of graph   Titles are placed below the graph. All graphs should use the term Figure (should be abbreviated to 'Fig.' rather than graph). All figures should have a number (e.g. Figure 2.2) and an informative title. The informative title should be clear enough to understand what is on the axes and what is being displayed. When it is a mean graph, the sample size should be stated, and if error bars are displayed, then these should be specified whether they are SEM or SD. After the title there should be a short legend giving details about the experiment and any abbreviations used, including asterisks to denote the significance. If the figure is taken from elsewhere or adapted then the source should be included (e.g. journal, website, book). An example of a figure title is shown below.

> Fig.x: Mean ($N = 15$) ± SEM Changes in Lactate Levels in Athletes and Non-athletes Before and After a Marathon Run.
> * = P < 0.05

Axes   Graphs should have axis titles (with units). The axes should also be scaled appropriately with regular tick marks. For each axis look at the range of values and subdivide using the tick marks. If numbers are small or large, logarithmic scales may be needed (e.g. dose-response graphs in pharmacology). Graphs do not have to have axes starting from zero. Some graphs start from a higher value without showing the zero. If the axis starts from zero and there is the likelihood of a big gap to the next tick mark, then it would be a good idea to show a break in the axis (Figures 2.3 and 2.4).

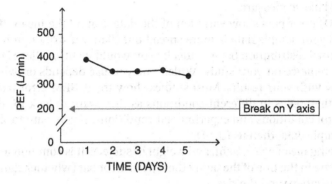

FIGURE 2.3   PEF variation on different days.

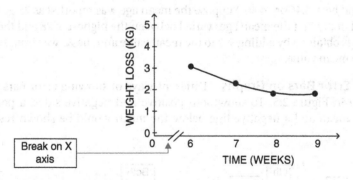

FIGURE 2.4   Weight loss over weeks.

Data Points   These can be individual values or mean values. Most publications show mean graphs. However, sometimes it is useful to show examples of individual graphs, particularly where an individual shows a different response from the majority (which may partly explain any variation shown). It is important to distinguish variables by different shading, colours or different shapes where you have multiple variables on one graph.

Error Bars Error bars are shown in mean graphs. They are a way of showing variation in the spread of sample data around the mean or variation of the accuracy of the calculated mean from the sample data. Typically, the data would be plotted with mean values plus error bars (commonly ± SEM or ±SD). The (±SEM) error bars give an indication of the error (accuracy) in the mean, i.e. the probability of finding the mean in the range given by the error bar (positive part of the error bar and the negative part of the error bar). The range of this error bar is determined by the sample data you have obtained. If the standard error bars are small, they indicate smaller errors in the mean quoted. Ideally your mean data should show small error bars for greater accuracy. Remember sample data can only give you an estimate of the population mean which is what we would like to measure.

The (± SD) error bars show variation of the data around the mean. If the SD is high it means your sample data is more spread out (flatter distribution in a normal curve; see normal distribution below). Ideally you would want smaller SD error bars to have more reliance on your study. Which one you use depends on what you are trying to show with your results. Most studies show the ± SEM error bars to show variations in the means in different conditions as they want to look for differences between control conditions and experimental conditions. If you want to show variation of the sample data, then use ± SD.

In describing mean age, height, and weight of subjects it is common to use ± SD. You need to state in the title of the figure the type of error bar (whether standard error or standard deviation) and the size.

The ± SEM indicates one standard error bar on either side of the mean (the error value would be multiplied by 1). The ± 2SEM indicates two standard error bars on either side of the mean (in this case you would multiply the error value by 2 for each side of the mean). So, if the SEM was 2.23, then in the plot the error bar on either side of the mean would be + 4.46 or –4.46. Suppose the mean age was reported as 25 ± 3SD years, this would imply that the mean ages varied between the highest of 28 and the lowest of 22. The 28 is obtained by adding + 3 to the mean value and the 22 was from subtracting 3 from the mean value.

Showing Error Bars on Graphs Different ways of showing error bars in graphs are shown in Figure 2.5. To show both positive and negative sides, a positive line above the mean and a negative line below the mean would be shown respectively.

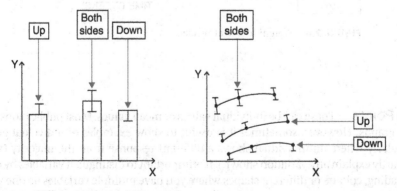

FIGURE 2.5 Different ways to show error bars on graphs.

Typically, when displaying mean data points, you show the error bars on both sides. However, error bars do not need to be shown on both the positive and negative sides. With mean bar graphs, the positive error bars are shown.

The size of the error bars displayed is a very useful judge of the reliability of the data. Large SEM error bars means less reliance on the accuracy of the mean and large SD error bars means wider variation. If you see that the ± SEM error bars overlap between two groups (e.g. a control group and an experimental group), then this indicates that the means from the two groups may not be different, and thus the two groups may be similar. This is important because usually from experiments we want to know if there is a significant difference in the means of the two groups, i.e. the difference in the means didn't occur by chance and can be repeatable. Hence, the means came from two different populations. To confirm this, you would have to do an inferential test (e.g. t-test) to see if the means of the two groups are the same or different.

The type of data will also determine how you show the central tendency and spread of your data. For normally distributed data you use the standard error and standard deviation. Data that doesn't follow a normal distribution could be shown using medians and interquartile range as in a box and whisker plot (see below).

How to Show Significant Results on a Graph   It is common to use asterisks next to a mean data point to indicate significant differences in the mean compared to the control (a difference not caused by chance). In Figure 2.6 the asterisk over the exercise bar indicates a significant difference in mean heart rate between control (rest) and exercise. The number of asterisks defines the significance level (see Chapter 3), with three asterisks showing a highly significant difference (highly unlikely for differences in the mean to be due to chance).

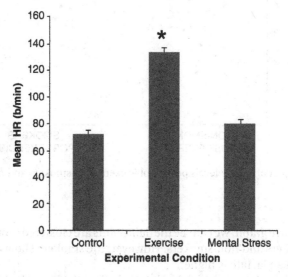

FIGURE 2.6   Mean (N = 12) HR ± SEM during experimental conditions; rest (control), exercise and mental stress. * = significant at P < 0.05.

The asterisks indicate the following:

*** = highly significant (P < 0.001)- chance of this occurring is 0.1% or 1 in a 1000

** = strongly significant (P < 0.01)- chance of this occurring is 1% or 1 in a 100

* = significant (P < 0.05)- chance of this occurring is 5% or 1 in 20

Types of Graphs to Display Data

There are many types of graphical methods to display data. These include: (i) dot plot, (ii) stem and leaf plot, (iii) box and whisker plot, (iv) scatter plot, (v) histogram, (vi) line plot, (vii) bar graph, (viii) pie chart, (ix) dose response, (x) Kaplan–Meier, (xi) Lineweaver–Burk, (xii) forest plot, (xiii) funnel plot, and (xiv) bubble plot. Examples of these are shown below.

Dot Plots

Also known as blob plots display each data point as a dot on a graph (Figure 2.7).

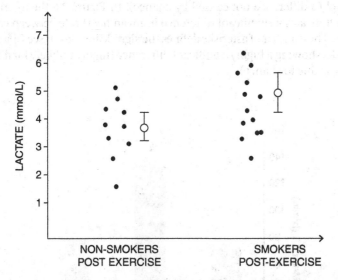

FIGURE 2.7 Dot plot of lactate levels post aerobic exercise in smokers and non-smokers.

From the above graph, we can see the data points are clustered around 3–4.5 mmol L^{-1} for both smokers and non-smokers. However, the smokers show a greater spread of values and mean lactate is higher.

Dot plots show the spread of the data (whether they are clustered together or more spread out) and show any high or low values. For a small sample (<15), a dot plot can be quickly produced on a line using a suitable scale (Figure 2.8).

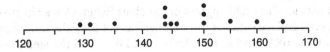

FIGURE 2.8   Dot plot of blood pressure (mmHg).

EXAMPLE 2.1 | Drawing a dot plot manually from raw data

The following systolic blood pressure values (in mmHg) were obtained from patients in a hospital ward:

    135, 150, 144, 131, 150, 144, 144, 160, 145, 166, 128, 150, 155, 146

Step 1: Find the lowest and highest values in the data and calculate the range

In this case it is 128 and 166 and the range is 166–128 = 38

Step 2: Draw a straight horizontal line and decide on a regular scale of tick marks to cover the range

---

A simple scale would be 10 mmHg intervals which would be represented by 1 cm lengths, i.e. 10 mmHg cm⁻¹. So, the lowest tick mark can be 120 and the highest will be 170. From the above plot we can see the spread of data, the lowest and highest values, that more data values are grouped around 143–150 mmHg.

Stem and Leaf Plots

These are used to display discrete and continuous values as a plot using the numbers themselves. The plot in Figure 2.9 shows 10 measurements of Haemoglobin (Hb) from 10 females.

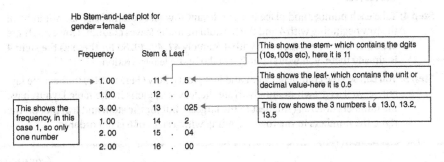

FIGURE 2.9   Stem and leaf plot of Hb in 10 women (from Chapter 8).

The plot may look like a histogram or bar chart (when viewed horizontally). The plot is based on the place value of the number, i.e. splitting the number into components of 10s, 100s, 1000s and so on which would be called the stems, and the units or decimal places would be the leaves. The values are split into two columns, one for stems and the other for leaves.

Each number is then placed in a row, based on the digit value representing the stem and the last number as the leaf. So, the numbers 12, 41, and 100 would have the stems as 1, 4, and 10 and the leaves would be 2, 1, and 0 respectively. If the numbers had decimals e.g. 5.4, 3.5, 20.4, then the stems would be 5, 3 and 20 and the leaves would be 4, 5, and 4. If you order your data from the lowest to the highest and then make a stem and leaf plot it is called an **ordered stem and leaf** plot. When you look at a stem and leaf plot, there should be a key (using one number separated by a vertical line) to illustrate the format of the plot. For example, 3|4 could be 34 or 3|4 could be 3.4. one of these needs to be specified on the diagram to clarify.

EXAMPLE 2.2 | Drawing a Stem and Leaf plot manually

At the end of a 1 minute reaction time test requiring the extinguishing of lights appearing randomly on a light board, the following scores of lights extinguished were obtained.

43, 47, 59, 54, 40, 65, 58, 55, 57, 60, 66, 52, 40, 35

Express the above as a stem and leaf plot

Step 1: Set up a two-column table, one for stem and the other for the leaves

Step 2: Find the lowest and highest values

We can see the lowest is 35 and the highest is 66.

Step 3: Set up rows for the digits, i.e. one row for the numbers beginning with 3, another for those with 4 and so on to 6. These would increase in order. Note, if there was a number missing for a row you would still put a row in. For example, if you had numbers only in the 20s and 40s, then the stem and leaf plot would have rows beginning with 2, 3, and 4, but the row containing 3 would have no numbers for the leaves.

Step 4: Take each number and place in the relevant row and column, e.g. 43, would be in the row beginning with 4 and the 3 would be in the leaves column. However, there are other numbers beginning with 4, namely 47, 40, 40. So for these as the stem 4 is already there, you would put 7, 0 and 0 in the leaves section.

Step 5: You can see the completed stem and leaf plots below (Figure 2.10) in the table layout, as well as drawn manually. Note the leaves sections in the table layout, have the numbers ordered (smallest to the largest), but for the stem and leaf plot on the right, the numbers in the row beginning with a stem of 6 is not ordered.

(continued)

EXAMPLE 2.2 | *(continued)*

Stem	Leaves
3	5
4	0037
5	245789
6	056

STEM	LEAVES
3	5
4	0 0 3 7
5	2 4 5 7 8 9
6	6 0 5

KEY: 3/5 = 35

FIGURE 2.10   Stem and leaf plots of lights extinguished.

Box and Whisker Plots

Box plots are used to plot groups of number data to show the distribution of a set of data usually in quartiles (dividing the data into four parts, see Figure 2.11). This can be used for smaller or larger samples. A box plot diagram consists of a central rectangle (the box) and two horizontal lines (whiskers) coming out from either side. The box represents 50% of the data, the lower whisker and the upper whisker represent 25% of data each.

Box plots show five terms which describe the distribution of the sample data. These are the **minimum value, first quartile (Q1), median, third quartile (Q3)** and the **maximum value**.

The central tendency is shown by the median and the spread of the data is shown by the quartiles and lowest and highest values. The **interquartile range** contains the middle 50% of the data when it is sorted into ascending order. It is the difference between Q3 and Q1 (also known as the 75th and 25th percentile respectively). Some data distributions may show **outliers.** These are data points which are extreme and do not necessarily mean an error, and they could be important.

Importance of a box plot

- Represents the middle part of the data as the median.
- Shows the variability or spread of the data by range, outliers, interquartile range.
- Indicates skewness, data congested to the right or the left or symmetrical.
- In publications box plots are shown vertically to visualize many data sets easily.
- Gives graphically a quick view of differences between different samples or groups.
- Indicates a difference between groups if the median is outside of another box, i.e. don't overlap.

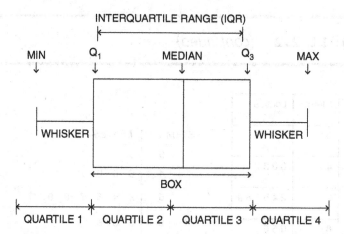

FIGURE 2.11 The structure of a box and whisker plot.

EXAMPLE 2.3 | Drawing a box and whisker plot from sample data manually

For a histology practical, the thickness of liver tissue sections in micrometres (μm) were:
7, 9, 3, 10, 12

Draw a box and whisker plot of this data.

Step 1: First order the data (smallest to highest), i.e. 3, 7, 9, 10, 12
Step 2: Find the median (middle number or 2nd quartile or 50th percentile), i.e. 9
Step 3: Find the first (median of lower set of numbers) and 3rd (median of upper set of numbers) quartiles:
Step 4: Calculate the 1st quartile (25th percentile) = (3 + 7)/2 = 5 μm
Step 5: Calculate the 3rd quartile (75th percentile) = (10 + 12)/2 = 11 μm
Step 6: Draw a plot line (scaled to cover the range)
Step 7: Mark 1st, 2nd and 3rd quartile
Step 8: Draw a box connecting the quartiles, then add the lowest (3) and the highest (12) values to represent the whiskers
Step 9: The completed box and whisker plot is shown in Figure 2.12.

This shows the minimum value = 3 μm; maximum value = 12 μm; first quartile (Q1) = 5 μm; Median = 9 μm; third quartile (Q3) = 11 μm;

An example of a box and whisker plot produced by software (SPSS) is shown in Figure 2.13. Note most publications would show this vertical presentation of a box plot.

(continued)

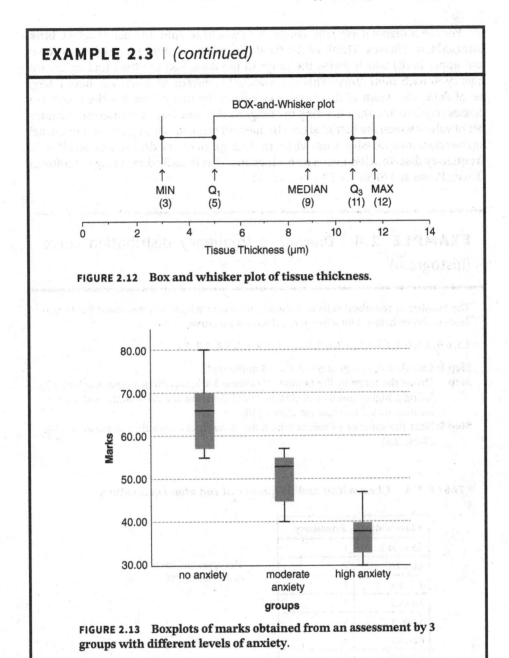

FIGURE 2.12   Box and whisker plot of tissue thickness.

FIGURE 2.13   Boxplots of marks obtained from an assessment by 3 groups with different levels of anxiety.

Frequency Histograms

Continuous or discrete data sampled randomly, are initially assessed to see the distribution of the data, i.e. if they fall into either a normal or non-normal distribution (see below). A frequency distribution curve (plot of frequency on the vertical axis against data or classes of data on the horizontal axis) would initially be drawn.

For the horizontal axis, the sample data would be split into bands called '**bins**', **intervals,** or **classes**. Think of the bands as groups of mini ranges (with a lower and upper limit) which divide the range of the data. You are then finding the frequency in each mini range. This is particularly convenient when you have a large set of data. The width of this band is calculated by first estimating the number of classes required and then dividing the range of the data. For each interval, the number of values which are included (the frequency) is noted. This results in a frequency against class interval table, from which the histogram can be drawn. This is called the **frequency distribution curve or histogram**. This is easily done using the software (Excel, Prism and SPSS-see Chapters 6,7,8).

EXAMPLE 2.4 | Drawing a frequency distribution curve (histogram)

The number of red blood cells in millions/microlitre which was measured for 15 students is shown below. Plot a frequency distribution curve.

3.5, 6.9, 5.5, 6.0, 4.3, 5.1, 4.7, 6.3, 5.2, 6.3, 5.9, 5.7, 5.8, 5.2, 6.1

Step 1: Calculate the range = 6.9–3.5 = 3.4 million/μL
Step 2: Divide the range by the number of classes, 3.4/7, this gives a class width of 0.5. Using a higher number of classes would decrease the class width and a lower number would increase the class width.
Step 3: Note the number of values which are in each class width and create a table (Table 2.3).

TABLE 2.3   **Class width and frequency of red blood cell values**

Class width	Frequency
3.5 <4.0	1
4.0 <4.5	1
4.5<5.0	1
5.0<5.5	3
5.5<6.0	4
6.0<6.5	4
6.5<7.0	1

The upper and lower limit of the class width

(continued)

EXAMPLE 2.4 | *(continued)*

Step 4: Plot frequency versus class width (Figure 2.14).

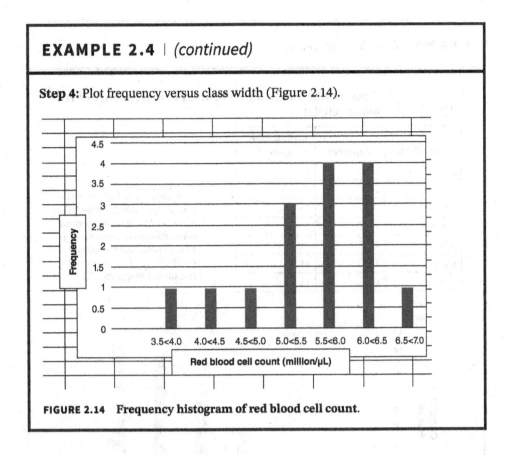

FIGURE 2.14   Frequency histogram of red blood cell count.

Cumulative Frequency Distribution Curve   Another form of the frequency distribution curve is the cumulative frequency plot (or **Ogive**) in which frequencies are added together and plotted against the class width. This is useful for finding the median, lower quartile and upper quartile range.

EXAMPLE 2.5 | Drawing a cumulative frequency distribution curve

Step 1: We will use the data from Example 2.4. First, add each class frequency to the previous cumulative frequency as shown in Table 2.4

Step 2: Plot cumulative frequency versus class width (Figure 2.15)

Note that the cumulative frequency could be converted to a percentage (Table 2.5) and then it is easier to find the median (50%, Q2), lower quartile (25%, Q1) and upper quartile (75%, Q3) values from a percentage frequency plot (as shown in Figure 2.16).

(continued)

EXAMPLE 2.5 | (continued)

| TABLE 2.4 | Class width, frequency and cumulative frequency of red blood cell data |

Class width	Frequency	Cumulative Frequency
3.5 <4.0	1	1
4.0 <4.5	1	2
4.5<5.0	1	3
5.0<5.5	3	6
5.5<6.0	4	10
6.0<6.5	4	14
6.5<7.0	1	15

Each cumulative frequency is obtained by adding the frequency of the next class to the previous class cumulative frequency e.g. 10 here is obtained by adding the frequency 4 to the previous cumulative frequency of 6

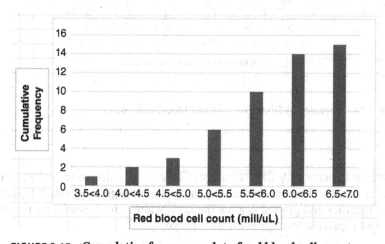

FIGURE 2.15 Cumulative frequency plot of red blood cell counts.

| TABLE 2.5 | Class width, frequency, cumulative frequency and percentage of red blood cell data |

Class width	Frequency	Cumulative Frequency	Percentage
3.5 <4.0	1	1	6.7
4.0 <4.5	1	2	13.3
4.5<5.0	1	3	20.0
5.0<5.5	3	6	40.0
5.5<6.0	4	10	66.7
6.0<6.5	4	14	93.3
6.5<7.0	1	15	100

Since total frequency is 15, then percentage is = (frequency/15) x 100-Here 13.3 is obtained from (2/15) x 100

Percentage Frequency Plot   Centiles are an alternative way of describing frequency distributions, where data is shown as percentages. E.g. 50th centile means 50% of subjects have this value or lower, 25th centile is equivalent to the first quartile, and 75th centile is equivalent to the 3rd quartile.

Another way of representing frequency distributions is to plot a relative frequency distribution where the relative frequency is calculated by dividing the observed frequencies by the total frequency. We could then replace the term relative frequency with probability (the chance of this happening), and thus read directly from the distribution the probability of an event, rather like the percentage frequency plot (Figure 2.16).

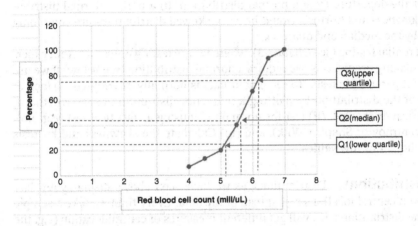

FIGURE 2.16   Percentage frequency plot of red blood cell count.

Types of Frequency Distributions   Frequency distributions (Figure 2.17) can be normal (symmetrical) or skewed (positively or to the right and negatively or to the left), where each distribution shows the mean, mode and median and the spread of the data.

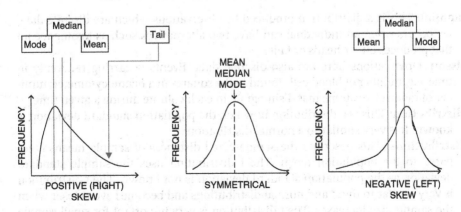

FIGURE 2.17   Different frequency distribution curves.

In the symmetrical (normal) distribution, the mean, mode, and median are all in the middle. In the asymmetrical or skewed distributions, the location of the mean, median, and mode will vary. In a right skewed distribution, the mean is to the right of the median and mode and most data is to the left of the mean (the 'tail'). In a left skewed distribution, the mean is to the left of the median and mode and most data are to the right of the mean in the 'tail'. Some data samples may show more than one mode in the distribution (for example, a bimodal distribution would have two peaks in the distribution representing the two modes).

Skewness can also be numerically stated with a number between ± 1. The closer the value is towards zero the more symmetrical the distribution, in fact a value of zero would give a perfect normal distribution. **Kurtosis** is a measure of how peaked or flat the distribution is; it usually varies from ± 3. The higher the kurtosis value the greater the departure from a normal distribution. In a perfect normal distribution, the skewness and kurtosis would be zero. Skewed distributions are commonly described by the median and quartiles.

In inferential testing (see Chapter 3), where we are testing outcomes from experiments by making predictions, we require a normal distribution (see below) if we use the powerful parametric tests. To see if your data is normally distributed, (i) look at the shape of the distribution by plotting a frequency distribution to see whether it is symmetrical or skewed, (ii) test for normality by using a statistical test (e.g. Kolmogorov–Smirnov or Shapiro–Wilk), and (iii) Calculate the skewness and kurtosis and see if they show low values.

Other Distributions

Distributions, as we have seen above, display your data showing both central locations and spread of the data. Every time we take a sample and plot the distributions, we will get different measures of central location (e.g. the mean) and spread of data (e.g. standard deviations). You would need to take large samples and many samples to find a distribution which equals or comes close to the population distribution mean and standard deviation.

Distributions are really a way of describing predictions of an event happening, i.e. we can think of them as probability distributions. Depending on your experiment (size of sample, type of data, design) we can make predictions about population distributions from our sample distributions by relating our sample distributions to established predicted distributions. Some examples of these distributions are as follows.

Binomial: This is a distribution produced by observations which are discrete data, i.e. occurs when an individual can have two alternatives such as tossing a coin that produces either heads or tails.

Poisson: Observations here are also discrete data. Events occurring randomly in time, e.g. number of blood cells found in the squares in a haemocytometer; number of radioactive atoms that disintegrate in each volume during a given time.

Z-distribution: This is a distribution in which the population standard deviation is known. It is very similar to a normal distribution.

t-distributions: This describes the standardized distances of sample means compared to the population mean. The t distribution uses the sample standard deviation as the population standard deviation is not known. The t distribution is very similar to the Z and normal distributions and becomes even closer when the sample size increases. The t distribution is very important for small sample sizes and is commonly used in t-tests.

Normal (Gaussian) distribution: The normal distribution (Figure 2.18), is the most popular distribution that you will encounter in biosciences. A large variety of biological data follow a normal distribution (e.g. height). So if we measured the height of a large sample of people and then plotted the frequency against height (where height is in classes or intervals), we would produce a normal distribution. If we know the population mean and standard deviation, we could easily plot the normal distribution. Suppose the heart rates of all students on a module were normally distributed with a mean of 70 b min^{-1} and a standard deviation of 5 b min^{-1}. This would produce a normal distribution plot as shown in Figure 2.18.

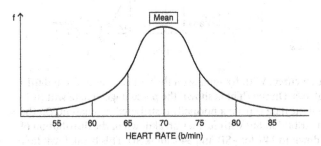

FIGURE 2.18 Normal distribution curve of heart rate with mean of 70 and standard deviation of 5 b min^{-1}.

This has a bell shape with tails that never touch the x-axis. The mean, median, and mode are at the same value. There is the same shape on either side of the mean (symmetrical distribution about the mean). The area under the curve is proportional to the number of observations, and since the curve is symmetrical, the area on either side of the mean is the same. The larger the sample, the more likely it is that they would show a normal distribution. The criteria for this distribution is that the data are continuous and values are drawn randomly from the population.

The centre of the distribution is the mean. The width of the distribution is

Normal Distribution

- Most important distribution in statistics.
- Most biological data affected by many factors tend to follow a normal distribution.
- It is a symmetrical (bell shape), with mean = mode = median in the centre, area under curve represents probability.
- Parametric tests require data to show a normal distribution.
- Normality can be checking the shape as a frequency histogram, or by analysis with tests of normality.

described by the standard deviation (SD), or how much the measurements differ from the mean, i.e. variability around the mean. In a large sample of data (>30) obtained from a normally distributed population, 68% of observations are within 1 SD; 95% are within 2 SD and 99.7% are within 3 SD (Figure 2.19). The area under the curve is 1(100%) and encloses the population.

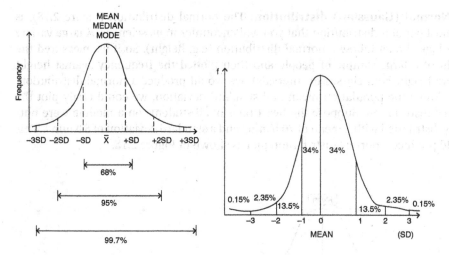

FIGURE 2.19 Normal distribution curve. With frequency on the vertical axis and standard deviation (SD) on the horizontal axis. On the right is shown the percentage of data within 1 (68%), 2 (95%) and 3 (99.7%) SD if the data is from a normally distributed population. On the left is shown the same normal distribution but with further breakdown of the distribution of the data, e.g. the 68% is broken down to 34% for –SD and 34% for + SD. This breakdown helps in calculations involving the normal population.

The advantage of knowing these percentages, is that we can predict the probability of finding a value or score. For example, there is a 68% probability of randomly finding a value between –1 SD and + 1 SD.

Z value (Score) and the normal distribution: The 'Z' score is a standardized score using standard deviations to describe

> **68-95-99.7 Rule**
>
> If your data is normally distributed (bell shaped)
> - 68% of data are within ± 1 SD.
> - 95% of data are within ± 2 SD.
> - 99.7% of data are within ± 3 SD.

how far away a data point is from the mean. It is also called the normal variate. Every sample data value can be converted to a Z score or value if the population mean and standard deviation is known, by the following formula:

Z = (X - mean of population)/standard deviation of population

Where, X is the sample data value.

If we plot the frequency of the Z scores against the standard deviation, we produce a distribution called the standard normal distribution with a mean of zero. This distribution of Z scores, allow the area or percentage to be found under a normal curve.

EXAMPLE 2.6 | Use of normal distribution and Z scores to solve problems

If the birth weights of babies were normally distributed, with a mean of 3.3 kg and a standard deviation of 0.5 kg, what is the percentage of babies born under 2.5 kg?

Answer:

Figure 2.20 shows the data for example 2.6 as a mean line drawn in the centre of the normal curve with a value of 3.3 kg and a line drawn for the data point of 2.5 kg.

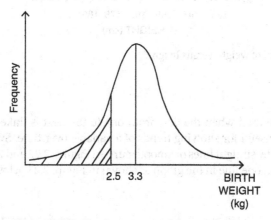

FIGURE 2.20   Normal distribution curve with population mean and data value.

Step 1: Find the value of the Z score

$$Z = (X\text{-mean})/SD$$
$$\text{Or } Z = (2.5\text{–}3.3)/0.5$$
$$\text{Or } Z = -1.6$$

Step 2: Using a Z score table (with negative values) look up the area for $Z = -1.6$
The area is 0.0548, thus the percentage of babies born under 2.5 kg is 54.8%

Scatter Plots

These are used to show the relationship between two continuous variables (Figure 2.21). The advantages include, (i) they show association between two variables, (ii) they use actual data values, (iii) outliers can be seen more clearly. The disadvantages include, (i) a weak relationship may not be apparent, (ii) difficult to visualize individual data amongst so many other data values.

They are commonly used for fitting standard curves in spectrophotometric assays, or to fit curves or straight lines to experimental points. The degree of association is found from doing a correlation test (see Chapter 4) and then finding the correlation coefficient, *r*.

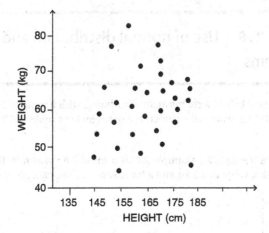

FIGURE 2.21 Scatter plot of weight versus height.

Line Graphs

Line graphs would be used when the data from one to the next is linked (e.g. changes with time). They are useful for showing trends of a variable over time. Symbols used for data points are joined by straight lines or smooth curves (Figures 2.22 and 2.23). Some line graphs have more than one line in the graph as shown in Figure 2.23 below.

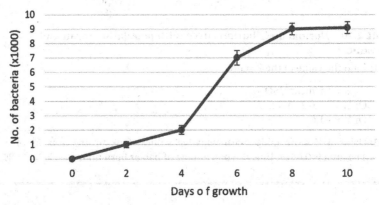

FIGURE 2.22 Bacterial number(±SD) versus days of growth.

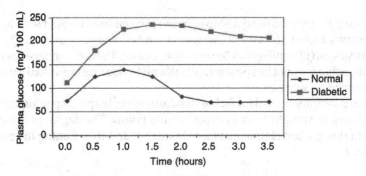

FIGURE 2.23 Glucose tolerance test with normal and diabetic patients.

Bar Graphs

Bar graphs show variables as rectangles either in the vertical or horizontal directions. Bar graphs would be used when there is no link between the data points (e.g. different conditions). Figure 2.24 shows a multiple bar graph of mean blood pressure changes in 10 subjects who were measured in four conditions. There were two control or baseline conditions (control 1 and control 2). The interventions were isometric exercise (HG) and isometric exercise with an ice pack at 0°C (HiAce). For each condition, the systolic (SP), diastolic (DP) and mean arterial pressure (MAP) were measured.

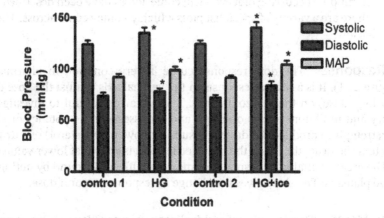

FIGURE 2.24   Mean (N = 10) ± SEM systolic, diastolic,MAP versus conditions. systolic = systolic pressure, Diastolic = diastolic pressure, MAP = mean arterial pressure, HG = handgrip, HG + ice = handgrip + ice. * = P < 0.05.

Pie Charts

These show data in a circle divided into slices (Figure 2.25). Each slice is a different category. The size of the slice represents the proportion or relative frequency of that category. It is used to display categorical data, data which show groups or categories (e.g. race, eye colour, blood groups, gender, religion).

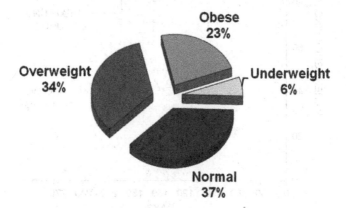

FIGURE 2.25   Proportion of women in England in different BMI categories.

Sections of the data all add up to a total value for a variable. In the example shown here, the pie chart shows the proportions of women in the UK in different BMI (body mass index) categories. The sum of all values should be 100%. Where the actual values are important, the % can be replaced with actual values. The advantage is that categories are shown very clearly. One disadvantage is if there are too many categories, then it is difficult to see all the categories clearly.

Other Types of Plots

The most commonly occurring plots you will come across have been described above. However, there are a variety of specialist plots which you may come across. These are described below.

Dose Response　The dose response curve is very common in pharmacology (see Figure 2.31). It is a plot of response on the vertical axis against the dose of drug (usually $\log_{10}$ dose) on the horizontal axis. These are very useful to investigate the excitatory and inhibitory effects of drugs, and for assessing the potency or efficacy (ability/strength to produce the desired result, e.g. lower cholesterol) of a drug. The more potent the drug, the lower the dose needed and is shown at lower values of the x axis. The greatest attainable response or maximal efficacy is found by noting when the curve plateaus. The slope gives the change in response per unit dose.

Kaplan–Meier　This is a plot of survival against time (Figure 2.26). It was proposed in 1958 by Edward Kaplan and Paul Meier to describe the probability of survival at different time intervals. It is typically used in clinical studies to monitor patients who have been given different treatments and their survival or onset to developing a side effect is measured. For example, you might compare a new drug against an existing drug in patients with diabetes.

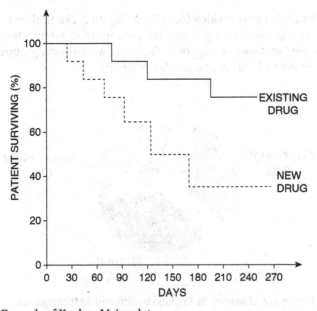

FIGURE 2.26　Example of Kaplan–Meier plot.

Lineweaver–Burk   This is a plot used to investigate enzyme kinetics (e.g. the inhibition of an enzyme), particularly in biochemical reactions. An enzyme is a protein which acts on a substance (substrate) to speed up chemical reactions. It is a graphical representation of the Lineweaver–Burk equation of enzyme kinetics, described by Hans Lineweaver and Dean Burk in 1934. It is a linear plot (Figure 2.27) of the reciprocal (inverse) of velocity (1/velocity) against reciprocal of the substrate concentration (1/substrate concentration). Its advantage is that you can obtain the strength of binding between an enzyme and its substrate (by finding K_m) and the maximum reaction velocity (V_{max}).

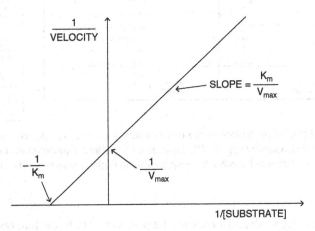

FIGURE 2.27   Example of Lineweaver–Burk plot.

Forest (Blobbogram)   This is a plot used to compare the results of several studies investigating a common aim. The name 'forest' was applied to the plot because a typical plot looked like a forest of lines. It is a standard plot produced in **meta-analysis** (which is a statistical analysis that combines the results of multiple studies (scientific or clinical) investigating the same aim).

Meta-analysis calculates: (i) the effect from each study (as an odds ratio or relative risk) and (ii) overall treatment effect as a weighted average of the individual summary statistics from each study. The **odds ratio** is a measure of effect size or experimental effect. It is the ratio of the probability of an event happening against the probability of it not happening. The **risk ratio** is the probability or risk of one outcome compared to the risk of another.

The plot (Figure 2.28) is laid out in three parts, with the middle part separated by a vertical line. This line is called the line of no effect (no clear difference between control and intervention groups). The left of the vertical line shows the included studies. For each included study there is a horizontal line (as a confidence interval). The middle part shows the results of the studies. If the horizontal lines cross the vertical line then there is no significant difference, but if it doesn't cross the line then there is a significant difference between the control and intervention. The diamond shape is the representation of the pooled result from the included studies. To the right of the vertical line the weighting (contribution) of each study to the pooled result is shown as a percentage. The bigger the sample size of the study, the narrower the confidence

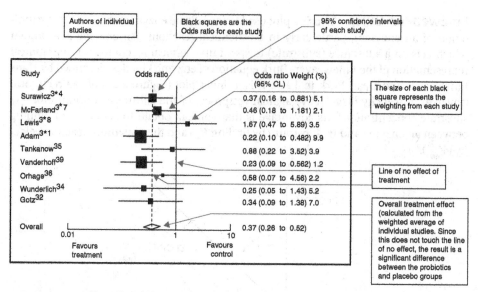

FIGURE 2.28 Effect of probiotics on the risk of antibiotic associated diarrhoea (from D'Souza et al 2002). *Source: Higgins JPT, Thomas J, Chandler J, Cumpston M, Li T, Page MJ, Welch VA (2019). Cochrane Handbook for Systematic Reviews of Interventions. 2nd Edition. Chichester (UK)*

interval and the bigger the influence on the pooled result. If the diamond touches the vertical line, then the overall pooled result is not significant.

The advantage of a forest plot is that it gives you the combined result from the pooled studies and it takes into account differences in size, methodology and results of the individual studies. The disadvantage is that the plot does not indicate publication bias (missing studies). This publication bias can be observed if a funnel plot is drawn (Figure 2.29).

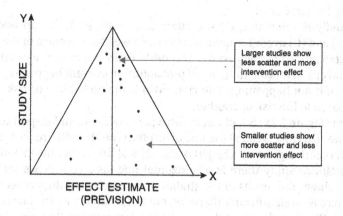

FIGURE 2.29 Example of funnel plot.

Funnel   This is a scatter plot of study size on the vertical axis against some measure of the study effect or precision. Note this is opposite to the normal plotting of effect or outcome of intervention on the vertical axis and variable being manipulated (in this case, study size) on the horizontal axis.

The shape is typically a pyramid (inverted funnel) and individual dots represent the different studies. The funnel shape is due to there being more small studies than large studies. They are useful for investigating publication bias (more large studies with significant results are published than small studies with non-significant results) in meta-analysis. A more pyramidal or funnel shape shows less publication bias.

Bubble   This is like a scatter plot (Figure 2.30), where the data is shown as bubbles. But, in addition the size of each data point is shown by the size of the bubble. It looks at the relationship between three numerical variables. If the sample size is high, then it is difficult to distinguish the data points which is also the same problem in other scatter plots.

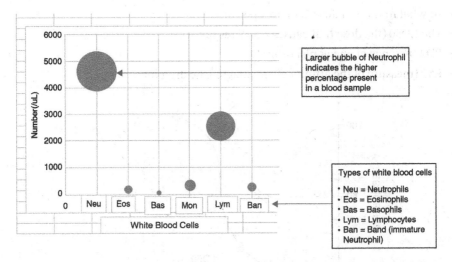

FIGURE 2.30   Example of bubble plot showing number of white blood cells versus type of white bood cell. Size of bubbles represent the % present in healthy adult.

Extracting Information from Graphs

Some common information obtained from graphs are shown below.

Relationship between the two variables

Calibration graphs are typically linear and very important in checking the accuracy of an instrument or for assays. Typically known values of 'X' would be put into the instrument and the 'Y' values would be recorded. From a plot of 'Y' versus 'X' a typical linear plot is expected, e.g. absorbance against concentration plot, from which the concentration of an unknown solution can be found.

Measurement of slope

The slope or gradient can be useful in finding the rate of change, e.g. a slope from a graph of oxygen uptake in mls versus time in minutes would give the rate of oxygen consumption in ml min^{-1}; or rate of enzyme reaction in a Michaelis Menten graph; to find the slope manually, a large right angle triangle would be drawn against the line and slope = height/base; slope in a linear relationship of the form $y = mx + c$ produced by Excel, would be given by 'm'.

Measurement of values from *x* axis or *y* axis intercepts

A dose response graph shows the relationship between the effect of a drug and the dose of drug given. Consider the dose–response curve shown in Figure 2.31. On the vertical axis we have the response in percentage and on the horizontal axis we have the dose in mg. From this we might want to calculate

- At what minimum dose is there a response.
- The LD50 (the dose that causes a 50% response).
- PD2 (potency of an agonist drug).
- PA2 (measure of the affinity of an antagonistic drug for a receptor).

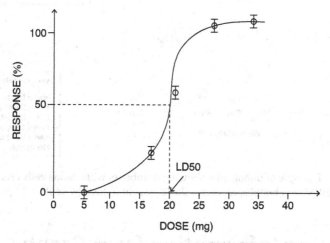

FIGURE 2.31   Dose response curve.

Summary

- Data can be displayed in tables with a table number and title at the top of table. Data shown as raw data and calculated descriptive statistical data.
- Data can be displayed graphically by a variety of graphs (dot plot, box and whisker, line plots, bar graphs, scatter plots, histograms), with a figure number and title at the bottom of graph.

- Typically graphs are shown with the dependent variable on the y axis and independent variable on the x axis.
- Raw data (each individual data value) are best shown in dot plots, stem and leaf and scatter plots.
- Box and whisker plots are very useful to show the central (median, inter-quartile range) and spread of data (minimum, maximum, lower quartile and upper quartiles). Can also show outliers and skewness of the data.
- Line graphs are useful to see changes of variables with time.
- Bar graphs are useful to show different groups or conditions (usually not related to time).
- A frequency distribution is a plot of frequency against data (grouped into intervals or classes).
- A normal distribution is a symmetrical or bell shaped frequency distribution curve, with mean, median and mode at the centre. It is important to show sample data follows this distribution if you want to use the powerful parametric tests.
- Error bars are used to show the uncertainty of finding the mean (standard error) or the variation of the data (standard deviation).
- Common information calculated from graphs are the slope, the intercept on the y axis, intercepts on x axis, r value (degree of relationship between two variables).

Sample Problems

1) A skin calliper was used to measure skinfold thickness in mm, at four sites on the body (superilliac, subscapula, biceps, and triceps) in four students . Three measurements were taken at each site. Using the following data create a table to display the data. In the table show the raw data and the descriptive statistics.

Student 1 (age 18 yrs, male), student 2 (age 19 yrs, male), student 3 (age 18.5 yrs, female), student 4 (age 21 yrs, female)

Superilliac: student 1 (5.2, 5.4, 5.8), student 2 (7.1, 7.8, 8.4), student 3 (10.4, 11.0, 11.9), student 4 (12.3, 13.5, 15.5)

Subscapula: student 1(7.1, 7.7, 8.0), student 2 (6.5, 8, 7.1), student 3 (8.4, 8.7, 9.0), student 4 (8.5, 10.5, 9.3)

Biceps: student 1(3.2, 2.3, 1.8), student 2 (3.0, 4.1, 3.5), student 3 (5.4, 5.7, 6), student 4 (3.2,4.3,4.1)

Triceps: student 1(4.5, 5.5, 4.0), student 2 (5.9, 4.8, 5.6), student 3 (7.8, 7.2, 7.9), student 4 (5.8, 6.5, 7.8)

2) Given the following absorbances and concentrations for a compound, draw a calibration graph. What is the concentration of x given the absorbance of x is 0.653

Concentration (mM)	0	0.5	1.0	1.5	2.0	2.5
Absorbance	0	0.173	0.349	0.521	0.692	0.864

3) The size of red blood cells in μm were measured using a microscope and graticule. Create (i) an ordered stem and leaf plot of the following data, and (ii) a box and whisker plot

7.8, 4.5, 6.7, 7.4, 8.5, 3.9, 6.4, 7.8, 6.3

4) From the following data of heights (in metres) of students, using suitable class intervals, draw a frequency histogram and comment on the shape of the distribution.

1.49, 1.53, 1.76, 1.72, 1.61, 1.77, 1.67, 1.55, 1.62, 1.85, 1.72, 1.70, 1.79, 1.79, 1.76, 1.79, 1.82, 1.84, 1.58, 1.84 1.62, 1.67, 1.69, 1.70, 1.73, 1.52, 1.60, 1.62, 1.71, 1.64, 1.57, 1.79

5) The following mean levels of iodine concentration (μg ml^{-1}) were measured in three food products. Plot a bar graph to display the data.

Cows milk: 320 ± SEM 20

Soya milk: 275 ± SEM 15

Seaweed: 194 ± SEM 11.5

CHAPTER 3

Choosing The Appropriate Statistical Test For Analysis

Expected Learning Outcomes

- Use hypothesis and significance in statistical analysis.
- Explain the importance of the P value, probability and confidence interval.
- Explain the difference between parametric and non-parametric tests.
- Choose an appropriate statistical test.

Having described the data by calculating descriptive statistics (Chapter 1), and by graphical methods (Chapter 2), we now want to analyse the data to answer the aims and hypotheses of our experiments. In most experiments, we are looking for differences in central tendency of our data (e.g. the mean or median), or associations between our data. Our prediction of what might happen is made in a hypothesis.

> "The null hypothesis is never proved or established, but is possibly disproved, in the course of experimentation. Every experiment may be said to exist only to give the facts a chance of disproving the null hypothesis."
> *Ronald. A. Fisher (1890–1962), British mathematician, statistician, Biologist*

Essential Statistics for Bioscientists, First Edition. Mohammed Meah.
© 2022 John Wiley & Sons Ltd. Published 2022 by John Wiley & Sons Ltd.

What is a Hypothesis?

> "The most important questions of life are, for the most part, really only problems of probability". *Pierre Simon, Marquis de Laplace (1749–1827), French mathematician, astronomer, Physicist*

Every experiment starts off with a hypothesis or prediction of what is likely to happen. We examine differences in the means or medians of sample data to either accept or reject a hypothesis. Or we examine the association between two variables to accept or reject a hypothesis as to whether there is an association or not. There are two main types of hypothesis.

Null Hypothesis

This states that there will be no significant difference between the conditions, i.e. mean of sample 1 = mean of sample 2. This is our **control hypothesis** in that we are saying there will be no significant effect.

Alternate Hypothesis

There is a significant difference in the means of the two conditions, i.e. mean of sample 1 is greater than or less than mean of sample 2. This is our **experimental hypothesis** which states that there will be a significant difference between conditions.

A significant effect or difference (see below) is a change that did not occur by chance, i.e. the chance of it happening is rare. This prediction of something happening is called probability and is crucial to accepting or rejecting a hypothesis.

Probability

To test the above hypothesis, we need to understand probability. Probability is the chance of something happening, it is defined between 0 and 1, where 1 represents 100% that it will occur (i.e. certain to occur) or zero, 100% that it won't occur. When we toss a coin there is a 50% chance of getting a head or tail (only two choices, heads or tails, i.e. $1/2 = 50\%$). However, if we toss a dice with six sides labelled 1 to 6, the probability of getting a number between 1 and 6 is 16.7% (six choices, $1/6 = 16.7\%$). To cover all the possible probabilities if we used 2 coins, or 3 coins or 50 coins we would have to do many experiments of tossing the coins to work out the frequency distributions.

Distributions

Historically (Appendix 1), probabilities have been worked out and frequency distributions (e.g. binomial, normal, Poisson distributions) have been produced from sample data (e.g. gambling). These sample probability distributions are useful in predicting outcomes and are crucial to hypothesis testing.

In Chapter 2 we looked at distributions of sample data, such as the frequency distribution and how the symmetrical distribution was equivalent to the normal distribution. From the population normal distribution, we could make predictions about our data (e.g. 95% of our data could be found within two standard deviations). So, if our sample data approximates to a normal distribution, we are testing the probability that our data came either from the same population or from a different population. To see if there is a difference, we need to do significance tests.

What is Significance?

In the above hypotheses, we are looking to see if the differences and associations are significant. What does significance mean? Significance refers to tests to see if differences occurred by chance. **If a test tells us that the result was probably not due to chance, the difference is said to be significant.**

Levels of Significance

The probability (P) value is used to determine if the result of a significant-test occurred due to chance factors. The P value is a measure of the probability of error in accepting the result of a significance test. The most common significance level set in statistical tests is 5% and is called the **P value of 0.05**. The smaller the P value, the less likely the difference in means was due to chance, i.e. rare event.

> **P value**
> - Is a probability value between 0 and 1.
> - It describes how likely your data would have occurred by chance.
> - It provides evidence to support or reject the null hypothesis: $P < 0.05$, accept null hypothesis; $P > 0.05$, reject null hypothesis.
> - Some statistical packages (e.g. SPSS) give P = -0000, this does not indicate zero, it indicates a very small number.

Suppose we want to know if the means of two sample groups are significantly different (alternative hypothesis) or the same (null hypothesis), then in our significance test we could use different P values:

if $P = 0.10$, then there is 90% certainty that the means are different between two groups

if $P = 0.05$, then there is 95% certainty that the means are different between two groups

if $P = 0.01$, then there is a 99% certainty that means are different two groups

if P is large, then the result is unreliable, the smaller the value the less likely the result was due to chance. If we find significant differences in the results, we can categorize these as follows

- Highly significant ($P < 0.001$): chance of this occurring is 0.1% or 1 in a 1000.
- Strongly significant ($P < 0.01$): chance of this occurring is 1% or 1 in a 100.
- Significant ($P < 0.05$): chance of this occurring is 5% or 1 in 20.

The most common threshold used for statistical significance is P = 5% = 5/100 = 0.05, which means that the significance level for the experiment has been set at 95% or P < 0.05. So, **if the P value obtained from comparing groups is below 0.05 then the result is significant** and if the P value is greater than 0.05, then the result is not significant.

> **"The probability is like the stick used by the blind man to feel his way. If he could see, he would not need the cane, just as if we knew which horse runs faster, then we would not need probability theory."**
> *Stanislaw Lem (1921–2006), Polish author of science fiction*

The Link between P Value and Confidence Interval

> A P value will tell you if you have a significant difference, but it won't tell you the size of the difference. A confidence interval will tell you the size of the difference.

From the above, we can see that the P value is used to tell us if there is a difference in the means between two groups and whether this difference is significant, strongly significant or highly significant. The P value does not tell you the actual size of the difference.

In Chapter 1, the term confidence interval (CI) was introduced. This was a measure of how confident we were as to the location of the mean based on a percentage level chosen for the CI. We mentioned that the most popular CI used was the 95%, i.e. we are 95% confident that the mean lies between a lower limit (mean –1.96 SEM) and an upper limit (mean + 1.96SEM). We can now relate this CI to the probability or level of significance by the following equation:

Level of confidence = 100% – level of significance
or,
Level of significance = 100 – level of confidence
or, substituting the CI for 95%,....
Level of significance = 100 – 95 = 5% = 0.05

Thus, setting a confidence level also sets the level of significance or P value. **A P value allows you to accept or reject the null hypothesis, it does not prove the null or alternative hypothesis**. A P value does not give the size of the acceptance or rejection of the null hypothesis. The advantage of the confidence interval is that it does give the size of acceptance or rejection.

Accuracy of the Mean

The advantage of the confidence interval is that it tells you the size of the difference in the means and the estimate of finding the population mean. The accuracy (or validity) of your study depends on finding an accurate estimate of the population mean. This accuracy is increased (i) if your sample size is high, (ii) if you took many samples, (iii) if your standard deviation is low, (iv) if your standard error is low, and (v) if your confidence interval is narrow.

An increase in sample size decreases your confidence interval which would increase your chances of finding the population mean. However, an increase in sample size may not always be possible due to cost. For example, in a clinical trial to cut costs, you may want to decrease the sample size of volunteers, but this would increase the confidence interval and thus reduce the chances of finding the population mean. A 99% CI has a higher significance level than a 95% CI, but the probability of finding the population mean is lower (more uncertainty).

Factors to Consider in Significance Testing

In carrying out significance or inferential tests (see below), the following aspects should be considered.

Critical Values

In addition to P values, predicted critical values (based on significance level and degrees of freedom) for various distributions are used to calculate significances. The critical value is a value obtained at a given confidence level (e.g. 95%, 99%), which is compared to the value obtained from a significance test. If you were doing a t-test, then you would compare the experimental t value obtained from your sample groups with the critical t value (for the degree of freedom and level of significance of your study). If your experimental t value is greater than the critical t value, then you are showing a significant result.

An example of using the critical value ($F_{critical}$) for the F-test is shown below in example 3.1. Statistical tables contain critical or predicted values at different levels of confidence. They show how large a difference needs to be before it can be considered significant. The software used to do statistical tests, show the critical values and even indicate which results are significant.

Two Sided or One Sided Tests

When we have two groups of sample data which have been obtained from a normal distribution, we can do either a one sided (one tailed hypothesis) or two sided test (two tailed hypothesis) for significance. The tails are the parts of the normal distribution on either side of the mean.

One tailed hypothesis This states that there will be a difference in a specified direction (only the area of one side of the normal distribution). In a one tailed hypothesis, the significance level would be on one side. For example, a 5% significance level would be either on the left tail or the right tail. A one tailed hypothesis is stronger, requires a smaller sample size but more difficult to show significance because the critical value to show significance is higher. The intervention is either greater than control or less than control. This type may be important clinically (one treatment better than another) or commercially (one drug is more effective than control). For example, a drug company which has produced a new antihypertensive drug (a drug which lowers blood pressure) may want to show if it works better than another existing antihypertensive drug. The disadvantage of a one tail test is that you cannot detect an effect in the other direction. Suppose you tested a new vaccine against an older vaccine and in your one tailed hypothesis you wanted to know if the new vaccine was better than the old vaccine. This can be tested, but you won't be able to tell if the new vaccine is less effective.

Two tailed hypothesis This does not specify the direction of the difference. Two tailed is much more common and represents the total area under the normal distribution curve. In a two tailed test the significance level would apply in both directions (e.g. a 5% significance level would have 2.5% in the left tail and 2.5% in the right tail). It is weaker than a one tail test because each direction is only half as strong. It is easier to show significance since the critical value to show significance is lower for a two tail test than a one tail test. For three or more groups a two tailed test would be used.

t-test

The t-test is a procedure to compare the means of two groups of data. It is a common inferential test which requires a critical t value to be superseded by the experimental t value in order to show significance. Critical value t tables for different significance levels are published that show how large a difference needs to be before it can be considered not to have occurred by chance (see Appendix 8). A two sample t-test assumes that the two independent samples come from populations with normal distribution and have the same standard deviation or variance. To test for similar variance between groups, we use the F-test (see below).

ANOVA (Analysis of Variance)

This is a test to compare the variability of the group means. It checks whether the variance is greater than would be expected by chance. It uses the F-test. The larger the F value the greater is the difference in the group means.

F-test

This test compares the spread (variance) of data between two or more groups.

F = variance of one group/variance of the other group

Usually larger variance on the top and smaller variance on bottom. It is commonly used in independent t-tests (to decide whether there is equal or unequal variance in the two groups). It is also used in ANOVA (analysis of variance) testing.

EXAMPLE 3.1 | Calculating the F-test to see if the variance in two groups are equal or unequal

Suppose we had two independent groups (N1 and N2). N1 has a sample size of 12 with a SD of 3.4 whilst N2 has a sample size of 15 with a SD of 4.2. Are the variances significantly different between the two groups?

Step 1: Rearrange the equation for the F value

F = Variance of sample N^1/Variance of N^2

Since, variance = square of the standard deviation (SD^2)

F = square of the standard deviation for N1/square of the standard deviation for N2

or, F = $(SD of N1)^2/(SD of N2)^2$

(continued)

EXAMPLE 3.1 *(continued)*

Step 2: Calculate the F value

$F = 4.2^2/3.4^2 = 17.64/11.56 = 1.53$

This is the calculated value ($F_{calculated}$)

Step 3: Calculate the degrees of freedom for each sample

Df for N1 = N1-1 = 12-1 = 11, df for N2 = N2-1 = 15-1 = 14

Step 4: Look up the critical value of F ($F_{critical}$) from the tables of $F_{critical}$ using df of 11 and 14 and the significance level of 0.05 (see Appendix 8).

The $F_{critical}$ value is 2.74

Step 5: Compare the $F_{calculated}$ and $F_{critical}$ values

Since $F_{critical}$ (2.74) > Calculated (1.53), then the SD comes from the same population, and we have equal variances in sample N1 and N2.

Errors of Significant Testing

There are two types of errors in reporting significance, one is a **type 1 error** (also called **false positive**), when we say result is significant when it is not, e.g. this can occur if we use the same data in repeated tests. The second is a **type 2 error** (also called **false negative**), the result is not significant when it is, this commonly occurs if the samples size is low.

Degrees of Freedom (df)

This is the number of variables (independent variables) that can be manipulated. In every significance test the degrees of freedom are important in finding the critical value for the distribution being used in the significance testing. Note the calculation for the df will vary depending on the type of test, but generally, df is equal to sample size minus one.

Tests of Normality

If we want to use tests such as t-tests and ANOVA, then we have to show that our sample data is normally distributed. To do this we can explore graphically by plotting frequency histograms or box and whisker plots or use tests of normality (e.g. Kolmogorov–Smirnov). If the data appears to be not normally distributed, then it is possible to transform the data and then repeat the tests for normality.

Types of Inferential Tests

We may want to know if there is a relationship between variables, and how strong that relationship is. We also want to know if there is

> "All models are wrong, but some are useful.
> Statisticians, like artists, have the bad habit of falling in love with their models."
> *Both by George Box (1919–2013), British statistician*

a difference between the controls and the interventions, and whether differences were significant or clinically significant (i.e. did the difference in the results occur by chance or is it a genuine change).

The questions asked are:

i. Are differences in the means real?
ii. Did the difference in the means occur by chance?
iii. Are the associations between the variables real or occurred by chance?
iv. What is the strength of the relationships between variables?
v. Are the variances of the groups the same or different?

These tests of significance are called inferential tests of statistics. The tests chosen will be determined by the design of your experiment and the type of data and the number of groups. These tests can be grouped into two types, parametric and non-parametric tests.

Parametric Tests
These are tests where the parameters of theoretical distributions (mean and standard deviations) are estimated, e.g. t-tests, ANOVA, correlation and regression. These statistical tests are used to compare differences usually in the means of sample data. They are powerful tests and can identify small differences. Commonly used with continuous data (e.g. serum cholesterol, blood flow, skinfold thickness).

Assumptions made for parametric tests:

i. Sample is representative of the population.
ii. Sample chosen randomly.
iii. Sample follows a normal distribution (data needs to be normally distributed, bell shaped frequency histogram (can plot a frequency histogram to see if you get a normal plot.
iv. Spread of data (variance) is uniform between groups.

If the assumptions are not met, then you might be able to transform the data and still use parametric tests or use the non-parametric tests.

Transforming Data Which Is Not Normally Distributed
Sample data which does not show a normal distribution, can be mathematically transformed to approximate normality. The most common methods are taking the log, square root, or reciprocal of the raw data. If the data is skewed (either to the left or to the right), then it may be possible to transform it to a normal distribution.

If each data was x, then positively skewed data can be transformed by taking the square root ($\sqrt{x}$), finding the $\log_{10}$ ($\log_{10} x$) or the reciprocal ($1/x$) of each data value. The most popular method is logarithmic transformation. Negatively skewed data can be transformed by squaring (x^2) or cubing (x^3) each data value. After transforming you would again plot a frequency distribution and test for normality. A lot of body size measurements are normal (e.g. height, weight). However, some blood parameter concentrations (e.g. K^+, creatine) may need to be log transformed for normality.

Non-Parametric Tests
Are tests (e.g. sign, Mann–Whitney, rank correlation) on data which don't follow a normal distribution. Skewed distribution data are often analysed by non-parametric methods. They are less powerful than parametric tests as (i) not all the data, or limited data, is used in the analysis, and (ii) they require bigger

differences in the data to show a significance. They involve ranking the data in order of the observations and then using these ranks in the calculations.

Inferential statistics (parametric or non-parametric- Table 3.1) analyse data to see if there are differences in the means (or medians), this is covered in Chapers 4 and 5.

How Do You Decide Which Statistical Test to Do

> "If I had an hour to solve a problem I'd spend 55 minute thinking about the problem and 5 minute thinking about solutions." — *Albert Einstein (1879–1955), Physicist*

Deciding on the inferential test or tests is not easy. There is no ideal method. If before the experiment, the design, the aim, the control and the size of the study were clearly defined then it is easier. If your study has some similarity to a published one, you can look at the design and statistical tests used and see how these could be applied to your study.

> "Would you tell me, please, which way I ought to go from here? That depends a good deal on where you want to get to. I don't much care where – Then it doesn't matter which way you go."
> *Lewis Carroll (1832–1898), English novelist from the book Alice in Wonderland*

Some of the problems you may have encountered are:

i. Subjects may have dropped out.
ii. Time to complete experiment was reduced.
iii. Techniques did not work so the protocol may have been altered.
iv. Final sample size was small.
v. Data does not follow a normal distribution.

Luckily there are some 'robust' tests (e.g. t-tests) which can be used even if your data doesn't follow all the assumptions required for a normal distribution, to use them or as mentioned above, you may be able to transform data so that it is normally distributed.

TABLE 3.1   Examples of parametric and non-parametric tests

Parametric tests	Non-Parametric tests
Student's t-test paired	Wilcoxans
Student's t-test unpaired	Mann–Whitney
One-way ANOVA	Sign test
Pearson Correlation (r squared)	Spearman rank correlation
Regression	Kruskal–Wallis
Two-way ANOVA	Analysis of variance by rank
	Chi-squared

> **"Divide each difficulty into as many parts as is feasible and necessary to resolve it."**
> *Rene Descartes (1596–1650), French mathematician, philosopher, from the book "Discourse on the Method"*

Another situation is which tests to use where you might want to explore subsidiary aims, besides the main aim. For example, if you had males and females in your group, you might want to investigate the effect of gender as a subsidiary aim. Here are some suggestions below and the summary flow (Figure 3.1) chart to help you decide.

Deciding on tests before the experiment

At the planning stage of a research proposal or grant application, you would have considered the design of the experiment. You would have had a main aim and maybe some subsidiary aims and formulated a hypothesis. If the project had involved humans or animals, your study would have been through ethics committees and grant bodies, which would have given comments on the statistical tests proposed. If it was a research proposal as part of a final year undergraduate project or masters or PhD, then you would have had feedback from supervisors. If you were lucky enough to see a statistician, then even better for confirmation of your intended analysis.

If possible, keep the design of you experiment (Chapter 1) simple (this of course may not be possible). Ideally, have one clear aim for the study, but if you have other subsidiary aims make a note of these. Clearly identify the control and the number of groups involved. If possible, calculate the sample size needed. Identify your dependent variable (what is it that you are measuring) and the independent variables (what interventions, experiments are you doing).

Deciding tests after the experiment

If you have access to a statistician or supervisor or someone who has more experience with statistical analysis, discuss the most appropriate test to use. You might even consider online forums, or online statistical websites or videos. I have suggested below some ways of approaching the task of choosing the tests.

After you have collected your data, summarize your data by doing descriptive statistics and explore the data by choosing suitable graphs (dot plots, box plots, bar, line) for both raw data and then for mean data with error bars (SD or SEM).

i. From the graphs decide on what questions you want to answer: are you looking for an association between variables (then you would be looking at correlation and regression) or looking for differences in the means compared to the controls (parametric and non-parametric tests)?

ii. Identify the type of data you have, in general if it is quantitative, lean more towards parametric tests and for qualitative it would be non-parametric. However, you need to break the data type down further into continuous and discrete and ordinal and nominal to make a better judgement.

iii. Look at your sample size, is this small (suggests non-parametric) or large (parametric)? However, you need to consider whether data is normally distributed. This is difficult to show with small samples. The smaller the sample the more difficult it will be to show a significance. If you look at the critical tables, the lower the degree of freedom the higher the critical value you must cross to show a significant result.

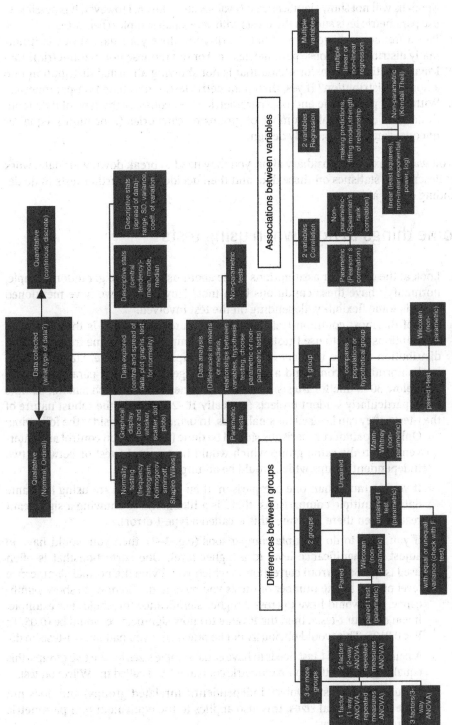

FIGURE 3.1 Flow chart showing the steps of data collection, data exploration and data analysis.

Non-parametric tests such as Mann–Whitney, Wilcoxon, sign, Spearman's and Kendalls will not show significance if N values are below 6. However, it is possible to use parametric tests such as the t-tests with very small samples (below 6).

iv. Plot a frequency histogram. What distribution does your data show: is it normally distributed (choose parametric tests) or not (choose non-parametric)? Can I mathematically transform data that is not showing a normal distribution into a normal distribution? If yes, then parametric test, if not, then non-parametric.

v. Within the parametric and non-parametric tests, consider the type of data (continuous or categorical), number of groups or categories (2 or more), equal or unequal sample sizes, study design.

If you want to explore subsidiary aims, you may need to break down your data, work out descriptive statistics on these data and then decide which further tests to do depending on the aims.

Some things to note when using tests

i. Look at the criteria or assumptions made about using tests (e.g. random sample, normality): have these conditions been met? However, as we have mentioned there is some flexibility, depending on the test involved.

ii. One of the most common tests used to compare two groups is the t-test. The assumptions made to use t-tests are that the sample groups come from a normal distribution and the variances of the two groups are the same. Statistical textbooks normally recommend a sample size bigger than 30 for parametric tests, but below 30 is fine for t-tests. A lot of experiments have much smaller sample sizes, particularly student projects (typically 10–20). Due to the robust nature of the t-tests, they can be used for small sizes. In using t-tests consider the following:

  o Only one pair of comparisons should be done (e.g. between control and intervention on the same group which would be a paired t-test or between two independent groups which would be an unpaired t-test).

  o If you do more than one comparison, then because you are using the same data in multiple comparisons, there is a likelihood of showing a significant result when there isn't one (this is called a type 1 error).

  o If you have to do multiple comparisons (e.g. 3–7), then you would have to adjust the significance level to a higher level. One correction that is often used is the Bonferroni correction in which you divide the normal significance level of 0.05 by the number of t-tests you have to do. So now, to show significance, you would have to cross a higher significance threshold. For example, if you did four t-tests, then the P value to show significance would be (0.05/4), $P < 0.0125$. This would obviously not be practical if you had many t-tests to do.

  o A paired or related t-test needs to have equal sample sizes for the two groups, this equally applies to the non-parametric equivalent-test called the Wilcoxon test.

  o An unpaired t-test involves independent (unrelated groups) and does not have to have equal sizes, this also applies to the equivalent non-parametric Mann–Whitney test.

  o If the experimental t value is negative, then only use the absolute value (i.e. ignore the negative sign) and then see if this value is greater than the t critical value for significance. For example, if the t value is –2.2, regard it as 2.2. See example in Chapter 6.

iii. ANOVA tests are the most appropriate to use when you have more than two groups. The three most common are one-way ANOVA, two-way ANOVA and repeated measures ANOVA.

- o In these tests you are comparing variances between groups and within groups to see if there are differences.

- o In choosing these tests you need to look at your design and decide on the factors involved. In one-way ANOVA you are looking at the effect of one factor on whatever you are measuring (dependent variable). This one factor is the independent variable, the one you are altering (e.g. treatment type (surgery, drug, placebo), exercise type, type of bacteria). Where you have to do multiple t-tests a one-way ANOVA would be the most appropriate.

- o In two-way ANOVA, you need to identify two factors. For example, you might be looking at treatment factor and time to recovery for patients. The two factors would be treatment and time. Suppose you measured the presence of bacteria in different locations, one factor would be type of bacteria and the other would be location.

- o Repeated measures ANOVA could involve one or two factors. It is like one-way and two-way, but since the measurements are repeated over multiple times (e.g. measuring blood pressure on the same group of subjects at different times of the day), this has to be considered in the calculations.

- o ANOVA tests indicate whether there is a significance between or within groups. They do not specify which pair of groups show significance. You would have to choose **'post hoc' tests** to identify which pairs are significant. For example, the Tukey and Scheffe tests are commonly used if you are comparing each group with all the others. If you are comparing a control group with the experimental groups, then a Dunnett-test is common. However, when you use the statistical software, you will have a lot more choice.

iv. Parametric tests are more powerful than non-parametric tests. So, if you have a choice go for parametric. Sometimes due to the low sample values you could be opting for a non-parametric test, but you may be able to do a t-test.

> **"Statistics are no substitute for judgement"**
> *Henry Clay (1777–1852), American lawyer, politician and skilled orator*

Summary Decision Flow Chart

Figure 3.1 summarizes the processes which we have mentioned above. As you can see, we have collected data, explored the data by summarizing descriptive statistics and displayed the data graphically. We then consider the data analysis which is being determined by whether we are looking for differences in the means or medians or looking for associations between variables. The specific tests (parametric and non-parametric) are then chosen based on the number of groups and types of associations.

> **"The combination of some data and an aching desire for an answer does not ensure that a reasonable answer can be extracted from a given body of data"**
> *John Tukey (1915–2000), American mathematician, statistician*

Summary

- Null hypothesis states that there is no difference in the means between two groups (control and intervention). The alternative hypothesis states there is a difference.
- Significance refers to tests to see if differences in means occurred by chance. A significant result means it did not occur by chance.
- Experiments set a significance level to determine if there is a significance or not in order to accept or reject the null hypothesis.
- A common significance level used is 5% ($P < 0.05$). This means there is a 1 in 20 chance of the event occurring.
- Inferential statistics use significant-tests to see if differences in means occurred by chance.
- A one tail significant-test is specifying the direction (i.e. an increase or a decrease). A two tail significance does not specify the direction.
- A critical value (based on degree of freedom) is used to test for significance. e.g. $t_{critical}$ and $F_{critical}$.
- Parametric tests are inferential tests used to assess differences in the means. They assume that the sample data comes from a normal distribution.
- Non-parametric tests are less powerfull and don't assume that the data comes from a normal distribution.
- In choosing inferential tests, you need to decide whether you are looking for differences in the means or associations between two variables. You need to consider sample size, type of data and experimental design.

Sample Problems

1) Two groups of patients who were diagnosed with a bacterial infection (Clostridium Difficile) were treated with two antibiotics (A and B): 5 out of 16 were cured with antibiotic A and 9 out of 12 were cured with antibiotic B.
   What test would you use to see if there was a difference between antibiotic A and B?

2) The concentration of nicotine was measured in a new E-cigarette by the traditional bioassay method and by two other methods, HPLC (high performance liquid chromatography) and GC-MS (gas chromatography mass spectrometry). Which test would you use to see if there is there any difference in the levels of nicotine by the different methods?

3) The effect of exercise on blood glucose levels was investigated in diabetics. A group of 30 people (matched for age) were recruited and split into three groups based on their glucose levels: a control group with normal sugar levels, a pre-diabetic group and a diabetic group. Each group then did one week of aerobic exercise or one week of high intensity exercise which was randomized. Blood glucose was measured at the end of each week after exercise. What test would you do to see if there was any effect of exercise on glucose levels?

4) Lung function was measured in 12 volunteers at rest and then repeated at three different angles of tilt. The angle of tilt was randomized for each subject. What test would you use to see if there was any difference in lung function at the different angles of tilt?

CHAPTER 4

Inferential Statistics

Parametric Tests

Expected Learning Outcomes

- Describe and calculate common parametric tests.
- Describe the principle of Analysis of Variance (ANOVA) tests.
- Explain the difference between correlation and regression.
- Recognise differences between parametric tests and their use.

Parametric

These are the most powerful statistical tests and are mainly used with continuous data. These tests are based on the assumption that sample data comes from a population which can be modelled by a probability distribution. The tests would normally expect a large sample size and sample data to be normally distributed. Parametric tests are able to distinguish smaller differences in means.

The most common parametric tests used are:

- Student's t (one sample, paired, unpaired, or independent).
- Analysis of variance (one-way, two-way, repeated measures, mixed design).
- Correlation.
- Regression.

More complicated parametric tests include:

- Multi-way ANOVA (multiple independent variables or treatments).
- Multiple regression (one dependent and multiple independent variables, i.e. one Y variable and multiple X variables for a Y against X graph).
- ANCOVA (analysis of covariance: looks at the differences and associations of slopes and intercepts of regression lines).

Essential Statistics for Bioscientists, First Edition. Mohammed Meah.
© 2022 John Wiley & Sons Ltd. Published 2022 by John Wiley & Sons Ltd.

- General Linear Model (investigate differences and associations, i.e. is a mixture of ANOVA and regression).

The common tests can be done manually, but the complicated tests are far easier to do with software. We will now describe the common parametric tests.

Student's t

The Student's t-test and t distribution were first described by William Sealy Gosset (who wrote under the pseudonym 'Student') in 1908. He was an English Statistician, Chemist, and Brewer. The t-test is a method of testing the hypothesis about mean differences in small samples drawn from a population which is normally distributed. It is a good test (robust) for looking at differences in the means for small samples. Its distribution is similar to a normal distribution (bell shaped curve). The test requires the calculation of the experimental t value (obtained from the sample data), and then comparing this with a predicted reference t value in tables (value determined by degree of freedom and significance level). If the experimental t value is greater than the predicted t value, then there is a significant difference in the means.

t = mean difference/SE of the difference

$$t = (\bar{x} - \mu) / \text{standard error}$$

or

$$t = (\bar{x} - \mu) / (SD / \sqrt{N})$$

Where t = t stat which can be + ve or –ve; $\bar{x}$ is the sample mean; μ is the expected value.

EXAMPLE 4.1 | Calculation of t for a single sample

Below is shown the data for 10 people who had their haemoglobin (Hb) in g/100 ml measured in blood:

16, 13, 14, 12, 12, 11, 11, 10, 9, 8

Is there a significant difference between the observed mean Hb and the population Hb reference of 15 g/100 ml of blood?

The null hypothesis is that there is no difference in mean observed Hb and the population Hb.

Step 1: Calculate the mean, SD and SEM of the Hb data

Mean = 11.6 g/100 ml; SD = 2.37 g/100 ml; SEM = 0.75 g/100 ml.

Step 2: Calculate the t value

t value = (observed data – reference value)/SEM of observed data

= (11.6 – 15)/0.75

= –4.53.

(continued)

EXAMPLE 4.1 (continued)

Step 3: Look up the predicted t value for 9 degrees of freedom and significance level of 0.05 from the t table (Appendix 8): thus t predicted = 2.262.

Step 4: Decide if there is a significant difference or not (if the experimental t value is greater than the predicted t value, then this is a significant result).

Here, the experimental t (4.53) is > Predicted t (2.262) thus there is a significant difference and the null hypothesis can be rejected.

Note: the negative sign on the experimental t value was ignored as we are only interested in the difference of the means.

Types of t Tests   The two most common types of t-tests are: (i) paired t-tests or related t-tests, and (ii) unpaired or independent t-tests. Examples of these are shown in Chapters 6, 7, and 8.

The Paired t Test   is used where the same group of subjects undergo more than one intervention or treatment in random order, e.g. control measurements (placebo) repeated by interventions (drug A).

t = (observed difference – hypothetical difference (zero))/SEM of the difference

The Unpaired t Test   The unpaired t-test is where the data is independent and comes from two separate groups, each subject only provides one set of data, e.g. exam results from cohort A compared to exam results from cohort B.

t = (mean of group 1 – mean of group 2)/ SEM of the mean difference of the 2 groups

This test requires variance to be considered, i.e. either with equal variance or unequal variance between the two groups (see Chapter 3). To check which test to do, an **F-test** is done to check for equality of the variances, i.e. the null hypothesis is that there is no difference in the variances between the two groups. The test involves dividing the largest variance group by the smallest variance group and calculating an F value.

F Value = larger sample variance/smaller sample variance

If the F Value is > $F_{critical}$ value, then the null hypothesis can be rejected, and the variances are unequal. If the F_{value} is < $F_{critical}$ value, then the variances are equal, and the null hypothesis can be accepted.

Note: the F critical value ($F_{critical}$) is obtained from a table of critical values (see Appendix 8), using the degrees of freedom of the larger sample and the smaller sample and the level of significance required (e.g. 5%).

Comparing Several Means

If we used t-tests to compare several means, there are lots of problems:

- Lots of comparisons to do, i.e. if m = number of groups, then number of comparisons is = $(m(m-1))/2$.

- More likely to be significant (type 1 error).
- Low degrees of freedom if groups are small.

To overcome these problems, we use ANOVA (analysis of variance).

ANOVA (Analysis of Variance)   The ANOVA test compares the variability of the data, within groups and between groups. It is used when three or more data sets are being compared. It compares the variance of each of the different samples. Variance is the spread, variation, or dispersion from the middle number (mean, mode, median). If two sets of data have the same mean and range, variance tells you which set of data has numbers more spread out from the mean.

$$\text{Variance} = \left(\Sigma\left(X - \bar{X}\right)^2\right)/N - 1$$

Or, SD = $\sqrt{\text{variance}}$.

Types of ANOVA

Randomized design   This is the variance from two sources, one source is within groups and the other is between groups

i)   One-way ANOVA: one factor or one treatment but many groups.
ii)   Two-way ANOVA: two factors but many groups.
iii)   Repeated measures ANOVA: member of a sample group measured under different conditions.

Block design   This is two relationships in the data points. Suppose there were three drugs available and you wanted volunteers to take these drugs at three different times, then each data point (say blood pressure) would be related by the type of drug given and the time.

Type of drug	Time		
	7 am	**11 am**	**3 pm**
A	X1	Y1	Z1
B	X2	Y2	Z2
C	X3	Y3	Z3

Calculation of ANOVA

In the calculation of ANOVA, our null hypothesis is that the means of the groups are the same. Our alternate hypothesis is that at least two means are different.

For the analysis we need to do four steps:

Step 1: Calculate variances within groups, between groups, and total variance:

i) Variance within (error or residual) groups (S_w): variation within each group, looks at how each value within the group varies from the group mean.

ii) Variance between (treatment or factor) groups (S_B): looks at how the mean of each group varies from the grand mean.

iii) Total variance (mean within and between variances) (S_T): this is the sum of within and between variances (i.e. $S_B + S_W$).

Step 2: Calculate the mean between group variance and the mean within group variance:

i) Mean between group variance (M_B) is the variance between groups (S_B) divided by the degrees of freedom (df)

ii) Mean within group variance (M_W) is the variance within groups (S_W) divided by the degrees of freedom (df).

Step 3: Calculate the F value ($F_{calculated}$) and compare with the $F_{critical}$ value obtained from tables or software:

i) $F_{calculated}$ = mean between variance (M_B)/mean within variance (M_W).

ii) If the $F_{calculated}$ is greater than the $F_{critical}$ then there is a significant difference between groups or within groups.

Note: if using software to calculate ANOVA, the results would be shown like Table 4.1, with the $F_{calculated}$ simply called 'F' or 'F ratio' and significance shown with a p value and a $F_{critical}$ value.

Step 4: Calculate which pair or pairs of variables in the groups are significant:

i) If significance is shown from the F value, then **post hoc** tests (e.g. Tukey, Bonferroni, Fischer's LSD) to find the pair which is significant.

ii) This is easily done using currently available software, with the type of post hoc test chosen depending on the type of ANOVA test used.

The advantage of ANOVA is that the effects of two or more factors can be examined, thus reducing the chance of a type 1 error. The disadvantages are that it doesn't tell you which groups are significant, also you have to choose carefully the type of ANOVA (one way, two way or repeated measures).

To do the above we need to calculate from the data (see Table 4.1):

- Sum of squares (SS),
- Mean squares (MS);
- Degrees of freedom between groups ($k-1$),
- Degrees of freedom within groups ($n-k$),
- Total degrees of freedom ($n-1$),
- Total variance (S_T) = between groups variance (S_B) + within groups variance (S_W)
- $F_{calculated}$ value = between group mean squares (M_B)/within group mean squares (M_W).
- **If $F_{calculated} > F_{critical}$ then reject null hypothesis**. The F-test is used to see if there is a significant difference between and within means of groups.

TABLE 4.1	ANOVA table. Where, k = number of groups, n = number of subjects, df = n–1, S_B = variance between groups, S_w = variance within groups, S_T = total variance (i.e. $S_B + S_w$)

Source	df	Sum of squares	Mean squares	F
Between groups (treatment)	k-1	S_B	$M_B = S_B/df$	$= M_B/M_w$
Within groups (error)	n-k	$S_w = S_T$-S_B	$M_w = S_w/df$	
Total	n-1	S_T		

EXAMPLE 4.2 | Calculation of one-way ANOVA manually using algebra

Consider in the table below three groups (e.g. these could be three different treatments (Group X, Group Y, and Group Z)). For each group we have three different values (for example the values could be days, blood pressure, size, i.e. X1 to X3,Y1 to Y3 and Z1 to Z3); the group means are $\bar{x}$, $\bar{y}$ and $\bar{z}$.

Groups	Group X	Group Y	Group Z
Values	X1	Y1	Z1
	X2	Y2	Z2
	X3	Y3	Z3
Mean	$\bar{x}$	$\bar{y}$	$\bar{z}$

Step by step procedure:

Step 1: Calculate the within groups variance (residual or error), i.e. S_w:
    a) For each group find the sum of squares:
        (i) Find the mean of each group (i.e $\bar{x}$, $\bar{y}$, $\bar{z}$).
        (ii) Subtract the mean from each group value,(i.e $(X1 - \bar{x})$, $(X2 - \bar{x})$, $(X3 - \bar{x})$; $(Y1 - \bar{y})$, $(Y2 - \bar{y})$, $(Y3 - \bar{y})$; $(Z1 - \bar{z})$, $(Z2 - \bar{z})$, $(Z3 - \bar{z})$.
        (iii) Square each value from (ii), i.e. $(X1 - \bar{x})^2$, repeat this for the other X, Y and Z values.
        (iv) Sum the squared values for groups X,Y and Z respectively.
    b) Add the sum of squares for all groups.
    c) Within group variance (S_w) = total sum of squares/df, where df = kn-k, where k = number of groups and n = size of group $S_w = ((X_i - \bar{x})^2 + (Y_i - \bar{y})2 + (Z_i - \bar{z})^2) / df$.
    where, X_i = X values; Y_i = Y values; Z_i = Z values.

Step 2: Calculate the between groups variance, i.e. S_B:
    a) Find the mean of all data, i.e. grand mean(M) = $(\bar{z} + \bar{x} + \bar{y})/3$
    b) Subtract the mean of each group from the grand mean
    c) Square the differences

(continued)

EXAMPLE 4.2 *(continued)*

d) Add the squared values.
e) Multiply by the number of values (n) in each group

$$S_B = \left[(\bar{x} - M)^2 + (\bar{y} - M)^2 + (\bar{z} - M)^2 \right] * n$$

Step 3: Calculate the variance of the whole data, i.e. S_T:
a) Find the mean of all the data ignoring groups, i.e. grand mean.
b) Work out the sum of squares for the total (i.e. each value – grand mean, square these differences, then sum of these squared values).
c) Then variance of total = total sum of squares/df, where df = number of total data –1.
d) Alternatively, $S_T = S_B + S_w$.

Step 4: Degrees of freedom:
a) Between groups the degrees of freedom = k–1, where k = number of groups.
b) Within groups the degrees of freedom = $k(n$-1), where n = number of values in each group.
c) Total degrees of freedom = nk–1.

Step 5: Mean squares:
a) This is a measure of the average deviation of individual values from their respective mean.
b) Mean square within groups (M_w) = S_w/df is the average variation within groups
c) Mean square between groups (M_B) = S_B /df is the average variation between groups.

Step 6: F ratio:
The F-test is used to see if there is a significant difference between means of groups
$F_{calculated} = M_B / M_w$
If $F_{calculated} > F_{critical}$ then reject null hypothesis.

EXAMPLE 4.3 | Calculation of one-way ANOVA manually

The FEV$_1$ (forced expiratory volume in 1 s) was measured in litres in three groups (each group had three people) as shown in Table 4.2:

TABLE 4.2 FEV$_1$ measured in normal, smokers, and obese adults

Groups	Control	Smokers	Obese
FEV$_1$ Values (L)	3.90	2.65	3.10
	3.65	2.40	3.35
	4.0	2.20	3.80

(continued)

EXAMPLE 4.3 *(continued)*

The null hypothesis is that there is no difference in the means of FEV_1 in the three groups.

Step 1: Calculation of group means and overall mean

Individual means = control $((3.90 + 3.65 + 4.0)/3 = 3.85)$, smokers $((2.65 + 2.40 + 2.20)/3) = 2.42)$, obese $((3.10 + 3.35 + 3.80)/3 = 3.42)$

Grand or overall mean $(M) = (3.85 + 2.42 + 3.42)/3 = 3.23$.

Step 2: Sum of squares (within groups) $= (3.9–3.85)^2 + (3.65–3.85)^2 + (4–3.85)^2 + (2.65–2.42)^2 + (2.40–2.42)^2 + (2.20–2.42)^2 + (3.1–3.42)^2 + (3.35–3.42)^2 + (3.80–3.42)^2 = 0.4184$.

Step 3: Sum of squares (between groups) $= ((3.85–3.23)^2 + (2.42–3.23)^2 + (3.42–3.23)^2) \times 3 = 3.2298$.

Step 4: Sum of squares (total) = sum of between and within groups sum of squares $= 3.2298 + 0.4184 = 3.6482$.

Step 5: Calculation of degrees of freedom

Df for sum of squares within groups $= k(n–1) = 3(3–1) = 6$

Df for sum of squares between groups $= k–1 = 2$

Df for sum of squares total $= nk–1 = 8$.

Step 6: Calculation of mean squares

Mean Square (within groups) $= 0.4184/6 = 0.0697\,333\,3$

Mean square (between groups) $= 3.2298/2 = 1.6149$.

Step 7: F ratio $=$ mean square between groups/mean square within groups $= 23.61$

From the F table, the critical F ratio is 5.14 (using 2, 6 df representing 2 along the x axis and 6 down the y axis (down the rows).

Thus, F ratio $> F_{crit}$

So, there is a significant difference in FEV_1 values in the means of the groups

Note: The one way ANOVA has identified that there is a significant difference in mean FEV_1, however, the test does not tell you in which group there is a significant difference, i.e. is it the smokers or the obese group which show a significant difference from the controls. To find this, a post hoc test needs to be done, such as Bonferroni, Tukey or Dunnetts. See Chapter 6 for this example calculated using Microsoft Excel.

Correlation

If two variables are related to each other so that they show a functional relationship between them, then they are correlated. It is a measure of the extent to which two sets of measurements show positive and negative association, i.e. the strength of any relationship.

Correlation can be positive or negative. The correlation coefficient (Pearson) is given the symbol r. This is a measure of the strength and direction of a linear relationship. This linear relationship is mathematically given as '$Y = mX + C$', where m is the slope or gradient and C is the intercept on the Y axis. In the figure below $m = 0.829$ and $C = 0.004$. Linear regression (see below) is a method of finding the best line of fit between the two variables.

The strength and direction of the linear relationship can vary from + 1 to –1. The closer the coefficient is to + 1 or –1, the more perfect the relationship; the closer to zero, the weaker the relationship. If $r = 0$, this means no correlation, $r = 1$ correlation is perfect (straight line produced), $r = –1$ means negative correlation. Generally, an r value > 0.8 is regarded as a strong correlation and a value < 0.5 is regarded as a weak correlation. In the calibration curve below $r = 0.98$ showing a strong correlation.

The square of r is called the **coefficient of determination** (r^2). In Figure 4.1, r^2 is 0.967. It is a measure of the variation (fluctuation) of one variable compared to the other variable. It is also a measure of the strength of the regression line for the two variables (Y on X). It represents the percentage of data closest to the line of best fit. For example, if r^2 is 0.90, then 90% of the variation in Y can be explained by the linear regression line Y versus X, the other 10% can't be explained.

It is important to note that showing a high correlation or significant relationship between two variables does not imply that one variable causes the other. It is also important to note that showing a correlation does not imply causation; further research would have to be done to prove causation. A classic example of this was the association between smoking and cancer which was suggested by some studies. This was proved by Sir Richard Doll and Hill (Doll and Hill 1950) who showed from epidemiological studies that smoking caused lung cancer and heart disease.

Another important aspect is that if a new method or technique or equipment was compared by correlation to an existing technique measuring the same variable (e.g. two methods of measuring oxygen) and show a high correlation, this does not mean that the new technique can replace the old one, since the correlation is expected as you are measuring the same variable. A method which is popular and still commonly used to show agreement between methods was proposed by Bland and Altman (1986) based on differences between the methods plotted against the mean of the two methods.

Use of correlation

i. To test the reliability or validity of a measuring instrument, such as a questionnaire or a selection procedure.

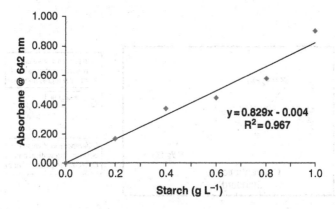

FIGURE 4.1 Calibration plot of absorbance versus starch concentration.

ii. To make predictions.
iii. To suggest hypotheses.

To use this test, the data must be normally distributed, the two data sets must be independent of each other (i.e. not be linked), only a single pair of measurements should be made on each subject and every r value calculated should be accompanied by a P value or CI.

$$r = \frac{\sum(x-\bar{x})(y-\bar{y})}{(\sum(x-\bar{x})^2 \sum(y-\bar{y})^2)^{0.5}}$$

$$= -1 \text{ to } 0 \text{ to } + 1$$

Degrees of freedom $= N-2$

The coefficient can be tested for significance, to distinguish between chance and consistent relationship. The larger the sample the better it is.

Regression Analysis

If two variables are correlated, then regression quantifies the numerical relationship, by using an equation. Regression is the method of finding an equation to represent the best fit line between the two variables. There are a variety of equations which may describe the relationship between the variables.

Linear Relationship Typically for a linear relationship a line of best fit is drawn, but this is prone to error if drawn by hand. The method used by software is called least squares method (Figure 4.2). This involves minimizing the distance between the points and the line both vertically (regression of y on x) and horizontally (regression of x on y). In effect we do two straight lines (using the equation of a straight line- $Y = mX + C$, where m = slope and C = intercept on axis), one is the regression line of Y on X and the other is the regression line of X on Y.

As you can see from Figure 4.2, the differences in x and the differences in y are used to fit the best straight line. The difference between the two lines becomes smaller as the points approach closer to the line.

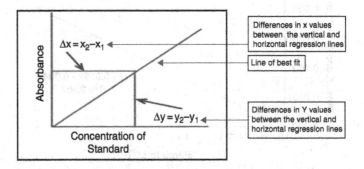

FIGURE 4.2 Regression line of best fit for absorbance versus concentration.

Non-linear Relationships When the relationship doesn't fit a linear model, then there are a variety of non-linear model options which can be fitted (statistical software packages give you a range of choices). Some examples include, quadratic ($Y = ax^2 + bx + c$), hyperbolic ($y = ((a + b)/(x + c))$) and exponential ($y = a^x$).

When there are more than two variables, there are methods called multivariate analyses to look for relationships between multiple variables. You will need to refer to other statistical resources to investigate these relationships.

Summary

- Parametric tests assume that sample data have been selected randomly and come from a normal distribution.
- Parametric tests are powerful tests which use continuous data and the actual data values (rather than ranking the data as in non-parametric tests).
- t tests are used to compare the means between two groups which can be independent (two separate samples).
- t tests are used to compare the means between two groups which are not independent (paired samples).
- ANOVA is a test to compare the means between three or more variables.
- F-tests are used to test for differences in variances in two (e.g. independent groups) or more groups.
- Correlation is a method to measure the association between two variables.
- Correlation can be positive or negative. The correlation coefficient (Pearson) is given the symbol r. This is a measure of the strength and direction of a linear relationship and can vary from + 1 to –1. The higher the value the stronger is the association.
- Regression is a method to quantify the strength of any relationship between two variables. Linear and non-linear models can be fitted to the relationship.

Sample Problems

1) Ten patients took a drug to induce sleep and the number of hours of sleep were counted. Is the drug effective?

Patient	1	2	3	4	5	6	7	8	9	10
Drug	10.6	7.5	9.0	5.4	6.1	10.2	7.1	9.7	8.5	7.9
control	8.6	7.3	9.4	5.1	5.4	9.0	6.5	7.9	8.7	6.9

2) Seven asthmatic patients were given two different bronchodilators A and B, on consecutive nights. Their peak flows in $1 \min^{-1}$ are measured each morning. Order is randomized. Does one bronchodilator work longer than another?

Patient	1	2	3	4	5	6	7
Bronchodilator A	340	550	400	530	410	358	425
Bronchodilator B	300	500	410	480	395	375	360

3) The number of yeast cells surviving after four treatments.

Tray	Number of yeast cells (per cm³)			
	A	**B**	**C**	**D**
1	27	38	29	19
2	30	40	42	27
3	38	37	28	24
4	30	36	29	21
5	32	41	26	23

Are there any differences between the four treatments ?

4) The following data was obtained of heart rates and ventilation measured with a metabolic analyser during exercise. Is there any association between ventilation and heart rate?

Subject	1	2	3	4	5	6	7
Ventilation (L min⁻¹)	22	40	53	64	90	135	160
Heart Rate (b min⁻¹)	103	110	125	138	150	165	177

CHAPTER 5

Inferential Statistics

Non-parametric Tests

Expected Learning Outcomes

- Recognise common non-parametric tests.
- Calculate examples of common non-parametric tests.
- Outline the advantages and disadvantages of non-parametric tests.

Non-parametric Tests

These tests are used with non-continuous data, when data is not normally distributed. They are often called distribution free tests, i.e. unlike the parametric tests they do not need the data to be normally distributed. Data are ranked in order, often small samples, and are distributed irregularly. It is the ranks that are used in the tests.They are often used to determine whether the medians of two sets of data are significantly different. These are less powerful statistical tests and need to show bigger difference in the means between two groups to show significance. Some common examples of these tests are shown below.

- Sign test.
- Fisher exact test.
- Wilcoxon (equivalent of the paired t-test): two sets of data of equal size.
- Mann–Whitney (equivalent of the unpaired or independent t-test): two sets of data of unequal size.
- Kruskal Wallis (equivalent of the one way ANOVA).
- Friedman test (equivalent of repeated measures ANOVA).
- Spearman rank correlation (equivalent of the Pearson's correlation test).

Essential Statistics for Bioscientists, First Edition. Mohammed Meah.
© 2022 John Wiley & Sons Ltd. Published 2022 by John Wiley & Sons Ltd.

Sign Test

The sign test was first introduced by James Arbuthnot in 1710. The sign test gets its name because plus and minus signs are used to replace data. It is useful when you can rank two values from a paired design (e.g. each subject acts as their own control).

This is a test to (i) compare differences between pairs of measurements
or (ii) see if the median of a group of numbers is different from a specified value.
It is used when the data is not normally distributed and is less powerful than the Wilcoxon test.

The steps to follow are:

Step 1: For each subject, determine the sign for the difference between the two values. If the subtraction shows a positive value put a + sign, if a negative value put a – sign.

Step 2: Count how many positive and negative signs there are and call this N. Suppose there were five positive signs and three negative signs, then $N = 8$.

Step 3: Note which signs are fewer and call this x. In this case $x = 3$.

Step 4: From the critical table for the sign test, look up the P value for N and x to see if it is significant ($P < 0.05$).

EXAMPLE 5.1 | Calculation of difference between pairs of measurements using Sign test

Suppose 10 subjects had their oral presentations assessed out of 100 on two occasions as shown in Table 5.1:

TABLE 5.1   **Oral presentation scores in consecutive weeks**

Subject	Week 1 score	Week 2 score	Sign
1	56	65	–
2	60	70	–
3	85	70	+
4	65	60	+
5	45	60	–
6	55	55	
7	68	75	–
8	62	55	+
9	75	71	+
10	63	60	+

(continued)

EXAMPLE 5.1 *(continued)*

Step 1: Put a + if the score is higher in week 1 and a – if week 2 shows a higher score.
Step 2: Count the number of subjects left after ignoring the subjects who show the same scores, N = 9.
Step 3: Count the total of the least popular number of signs, i.e. four negative signs, call this X.
Step 4: From signs predicted table look up the critical value for $N = 9$ and $X = 4$, this gives $P = 1$; since 1 is > 0.05, the result is not significant at the 5% level for a two tail test.

Wilcoxon Test

This test was developed by Frank Wilcoxan in 1945. It is a non-parametric equivalent of the paired t-test. It tests whether the median of the two data sets is equal or if data sets are drawn from the same population. It can be used with small samples and non-normal distributions. This test looks at differences in direction and size, unlike the sign test, and hence it is more powerful.

EXAMPLE 5.2 | Calculation of differences between two scores using a Wilcoxan test

Suppose we use the data above that we used for the sign test, this is shown in Table 5.2.

TABLE 5.2   Oral presentation scores in week 1 and week 2

Subject	Week 1 score	Week 2 score	Difference (wk1-wk2)	Signed Rank
1	56	65	–10	–6.5
2	60	70	–10	–6.5
3	85	70	+15	+8.5
4	65	60	+5	+3
5	45	60	–15	–8.5
6	55	55	0	
7	68	75	–7	–4.5
8	62	55	+7	+4.5
9	75	71	+4	+2
10	63	60	+3	+1

(continued)

EXAMPLE 5.2 *(continued)*

Step 1: Find the difference between the scores for the two weeks.
Step 2: Rank the differences in order of size (ignore the sign).
Step 3: Assign + ve and -ve signs.
Step 4: Find the sum of the + ve ranks.
Step 5: Find the sum of the –ve ranks.
Step 6: Using the N value and the Wilcoxan critical table (see Appendix 8) find the probability level at which the lowest rank value is less than or equal to the critical value, this means significance. If the lowest rank is > critical value, it is not significant. If one of the differences is zero then when looking up the table, use $N = N–1$.

As subject 6 shows a zero difference, it is not used in the rankings and N is reduced to 9 where there is a tied rank, the average rank is calculated.
Sum of + ve ranks = 19
Sum of –ve ranks = –26
Total sum of ranks = 45
Also, total sum of ranks = $N(N + 1)/2 = 9(10)/2 = 45$
Thus $N = 9$ and the lowest sum of rank = 26.
The critical value for $N = 9$ at 0.05 two tail, is 6, thus the result is not significant (19 > 6).

Mann–Whitney U Test

Is a non-parametric equivalent of the unpaired t-test. It tests whether the median of the two data sets is equal or if data sets are drawn from the same population. It can be used with small samples and non-normal distributions.

The test involves calculating the differences between results for two independent groups, group A and B. Firstly, the scores for each group are ranked, then these ranks are summed for each group, then the lowest sum of ranks are identified. Lastly, using the N1 and N2 values and the Mann–Whitney critical values table (see Appendix 8), check to see if the lowest sum of ranks is equal to or below the critical value for significance.

EXAMPLE 5.3 | Calculation of the differences in results for two groups using a Mann–Whitney U test

TABLE 5.3   Lab practical exam scores for two groups (group A and B)

Subject	Group A	Rank for Gp A	Group B	Rank for Gp B
1	25	1	85	10
2	72	7	63	5

(continued)

EXAMPLE 5.3 *(continued)*

Subject	Group A	Rank for Gp A	Group B	Rank for Gp B
3	56	4	50	4
4	60	5	72	8
5	40	2	65	7
6	45	3	76	9
7	65	6	18	1
8			25	2
9			64	6
10			36	3
sum		28		55
N	7		10	

The results from a lab exam were compared between two groups who took the exam in different rooms as shown in Table 5.3.

Step 1: Group A data was ranked from the lowest (25) to the highest (72)

Step 2: Group B data was ranked from the lowest (18) to the highest (85)

Step 3: The sum of the ranks for group A was 28 and the sum of the ranks for group B was 55

Step 4: The critical value for $N = 7$ and 10 is 14 (from the Mann–Whitney critical values table)

Step 5: Check for significance (if the lowest sum of ranks is equal or greater than the critical value), in this case 28 is > 14, thus result is significant.

Chi-squared Test

Is a test used to compare observed results with expected results (theoretical data). It tests for differences between categories within variables and looks for association (whether frequencies are related) between categories. For example, are infection rates different for people in different blood groups; do men and women have different probabilities of smoking?

Typically, data is put into tables called contingency tables (in a two way format) as observed and expected frequencies, and a chi-squared value is calculated. This chi-squared value tells you how much difference exists between the observed and expected values in each cell to the values you would expect if there was no relationship. The tables are filled in using the following calculations:

i.   Observed (O) values are given.

ii.   Expected (E) or estimated values are calculated from the column and row totals, i.e. E = expected = (column total x row total)/grand total.

iii. Degrees of freedom = ((number of columns −1) x (number of rows −1)).

iv. Then the chi-squared value is calculate using the formula.

$$\text{chi squared} = \sum \frac{(O-E)^2}{E}$$

v. If the chi-squared value is greater than critical value for the degrees of freedom and level of significance (obtained from chi-squared tables), then there is a significant difference.

EXAMPLE 5.4 | Calculation of the chi-squared test

Two groups (A and B) of a 100 each have a disease condition. A serum is given to group A, but not to group B: 75 people recover from group A, and 65 from group B.

a) Does the serum help in curing the disease?

Step 1: Set up a contingency table using the above information for observed

Observed	Recover	No recovery	Total
Group A	75		100
Group B	65		100
Total			

Step 2: Complete the box above

Observed	Recover	No recovery	Total
Group A	75	25	100
Group B	65	35	100
Total	140	60	200

Step 3: Use the formula for the expected frequencies to complete the expected frequencies box.

$E = $ (row total x column total)/grand total

Where the grand total is the total number of observations $= 200$,
e.g. for the value of 75 above observed for group A,
expected $(E) = (100 \times 140)/200 = 70$

Expected	Recover	No recovery	Total
Group A	70	30	100
Group B	70	30	100
Total	140	60	200

Step 4: The complete observed and expected frequencies boxes are shown below, calculate the degrees of freedom (df).

(continued)

EXAMPLE 5.4 *(continued)*

df = ((number of columns –1) x (number of rows –1)) = (2–1) x (2-1) = 1 (note if df = 1, normally a correction would be made to chi-squared formula).

	Recover	No recovery	Total
Group A	75	25	100
Group B	65	35	100
Total	140	60	200

Expected	Recover	No recovery	Total
Group A	70	30	100
Group B	70	30	100
Total	140	60	200

Step 5: Calculate the chi-squared statistic using the observed and expected frequencies
$X^2 = \Sigma\ [(O–E)/E]$, where O = observed readings, E = estimated readings
= (75–70)2/70 + (65–70)2/70 +(25–30)2/30 + (35–30)2/30
= 2.38
Step 6: Look up the predicted chi-squared value for df of 1, and P = 5%

Predicted X^2 = 3.84. Since experimental chi value of 2.38 is less than this then there is no significance. So, the serum does not cure the disease.

Fisher Exact Test

This is like the chi-square test for categorical data but for small sample sizes. This is used for two sample groups for two criteria, e.g. tumour cells present or absent; positive or negative; cured or not cured. Data is nominal (categorical, e.g. gender, race) or ordinal (scale data, e.g. pain scale).

Kruskal Wallis Test

This is the non-parametric equivalent of the one way ANOVA test. It assumes data samples are independent and groups have equal variance. The data is continuous data or ordinal data (e.g. Likert scale). Data is pooled and ranked. It compares whether the medians of three or more groups are the same. It is similar to Wilcoxon's or the Mann–Whitney test but for more than two groups. Differences in the medians are compared with a chi-squared test. If there is a significant difference, then the particular pair of groups are identified by post hoc tests. An example is shown using SPSS software in Chapter 8.

Friedman Test

This is the non-parametric equivalent of the repeated measures ANOVA. It assumes that data samples are independent and groups have equal variance. The data is continuous data or ordinal data (e.g. Likert scale). Data are ranked. Differences in medians are compared using a chi-squared test. One group is measured three or more times. An example is shown using SPSS software in Chapter 8.

Spearman Rank Correlation

This is the equivalent to the parametric Pearson Correlation test but is less powerful. It tests the relationship between two variables. The strength of the relationship is shown by calculating the r value.

EXAMPLE 5.5 | Calculation of the Spearman Rank correlation theoretically

---

Step 1: For each variable rank the scores (from the lowest to the highest). If two scores are the same, then average the two ranks. If more than two scores are the same, then sum the number of ranks and divide by the number of scores which are the same and give the result as the rank for to each equal score.

Step 2: Find the difference between the ranks for each subject (d).

Step 3: Square d.

Step 4: Find sum of squared d.

Step 5: Calculate r
$R = 1 - (6(\text{sum of } d \text{ squared}))/N (N \text{ squared} - 1)$
Where $N =$ no. of subjects.

Step 6: If R is equal or greater than r critical value, at the 5% level then the result would be significant.

Summary

- Non-parametric tests are used on non-continuous data which do not show a normal distribution. They are less powerful than parametric tests.
- Most tests involve ranking of the data.
- The sign test is used to test for differences between pairs of data, e.g. before and after treatment.
- The Wilcoxon test is used to show the differences between two groups who are related (this is the non-parametric equivalent of the paired t-test).
- The Mann–Whitney test is used to show differences between two independent groups (this is the non-parametric equivalent of the independent t-test).

- The chi-squared test is used to compare observed results with expected results in categorical data (e.g. race, gender).
- The Spearman Ranks test is used to show any relationship between two variables (this is the non-parametric equivalent of the Pearson's correlation test).

Sample Problems

1) Urine flow (ml min^{-1}) is measured before and after giving a diuretic. Is the diuretic effective in increasing urine flow?

   Before 2, 1.9, 2.1, 1.5, 2.0, 2.1, 1.7, 2.2, 2.6
   After 3.5, 2.3, 2.3, 1.9, 2.0, 2.2, 1.9, 1.9, 2.9
2) The blood urea levels were measured in two groups of patients (group A and B). Is there a significant difference in the urea levels?
   Group A: 28, 24, 39, 30, 32, 26, 27
   Group B: 40, 31, 33, 42, 35, 34, 38, 37, 46, 36
3) Eight histologists were asked to score two similar slides (S1, S2) out of 15. Are the marks significantly different between the two slides?

Histologist	Score S1	Score S2
1	8	7
2	10	7
3	12	9
4	9	4
5	15	7
6	12	10
7	9	14
8	8	11

4) Two patient groups, A and B, contain 45 and 55 people. Group A received the drug, group b received a placebo. It was found that 30 receiving the drug improved, but only 10 showed improvement in the placebo group. Does the drug significantly improve health?

Statistical Software Packages

Three common statistical packages which students will come across are Microsoft Excel, Prism (Graphpad software) and SPSS for both Windows and MAC computers.

The author recognises that other statistical packages are available, however, these were chosen for the following reasons:

- **Microsoft Excel** is widely available on most computers and is good for large data storage, analysis, and graphical presentation of data in science and business areas but limited in more advanced statistical tools, graphical display, and interpretation of results. It is good for parametric tests, but very little on non-parametric tests. There are a good range of statistical formulas but the use of these formulas and help and interpretation of results is weak.

- **GraphPad Prism** provides wider statistical tests (parametric and non-parametric), helps with interpretation, is excellent for graphical display of data, and is popular in the field of bioscience. It is interactive as any changes to data are shown graphically and in the analysis.

- SPSS is the most comprehensive is SPSS and the most powerful software package for statistical tests. Both parametric and non-parametric can be performed and is more widely applicable to social sciences and business but is fine for bioscience too. However, it is weaker on graphical display.

In addition to the information provided on using these in the next three chapters, there are textbooks, websites, and videos (e.g. on YouTube) which may also be useful. For the examples that follow, we have used Microsoft Excel (2016), GraphPad Prism (version 4) and SPSS (version 26). If you have different versions, you will still be able to do the analysis as the main structure and design is very similar.

Please note that in using statistical tests, assumptions or criteria relevant to that test need to be confirmed or assumed or justified. For example:

- Whether the data are normally distributed for doing parametric tests, if not whether the data can be normalized.
- Is the size of the sample appropriate for the test.
- Is the type of data appropriate for the test.
- In an independent t-test we need to check whether the variances are equal or unequal.
- In using ANOVA, we need to check whether the sphericity (variances between groups are equal) criteria has been met.
- Is the type of ANOVA test appropriate (e.g. one way, two way, repeated measures).

In the examples that follow, I have not shown in every example that these assumptions apply.

CHAPTER 6

Using Excel

Descriptive and Inferential Statistics

Expected Learning Outcomes

- Explain the structure and layout of Microsoft Excel.
- Input data into Excel.
- Calculate descriptive statistics using formulas.
- Analyse descriptive statistics using the 'Data Analysis' tab.
- Perform inferential statistics using 'Data Analysis' tab.
- Graphically display data using appropriate graphs.

What is Microsoft Excel?

Microsoft Excel is a widely used software spreadsheet for storing, analysing and displaying data in a wide area of fields (e.g. science, engineering, and finance). It is commonly packaged with other Microsoft Office software (e.g. Office 365).

The details shown below are from Microsoft Excel (2016) running on Windows 10. The spreadsheet is composed of cells arranged in rows and columns. Data (numeric or non-numeric) are put into the cells and then using the tabs at the top of the spreadsheet, the data can be analysed or graphically presented.

Excel uses data series (which is a row of numbers or column of numbers). These would be used for graphical plots and analysis. It is important that the data series have a name (variable name, and the data values are associated with this variable). The 'Format Cell' tab allows you to specify the type of data for that cell.

How to Input Sample Data

Data obtained (imported) from other software or typed in manually is put into the cells and tables (columns and rows). Tables are much easier with this software

Essential Statistics for Bioscientists, First Edition. Mohammed Meah.
© 2022 John Wiley & Sons Ltd. Published 2022 by John Wiley & Sons Ltd.

because a spreadsheet is already set out as columns and rows and they have the added advantage of using formulas to analyse and display data (i.e. statistical analysis and graph plotting).

EXAMPLE 6.1 | Putting data into an Excel spreadsheet

Step 1: Open Microsoft Excel, a spreadsheet with columns labelled with the letters of the alphabet starting from 'A' and rows numbered from 1 onwards is shown.

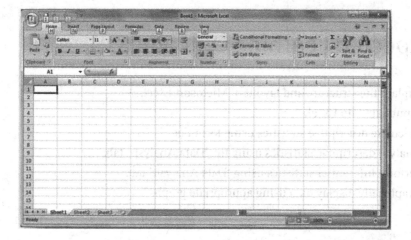

Step 2: Type the names of the variables in the first row with the units in the second row.

Step 3: Type the subject number or initials in the first column.

This column has the variable name 'age' in cell C1; units of 'yrs' in cell C2; the data is contained in cells C3 to C8

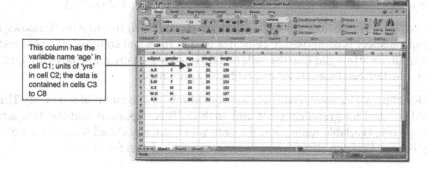

Step 4: Type in your data.

As you can see the data presented in columns and rows are in the cells A1 to E8.

Using Formulas to Calculate Statistical Terms

To use formulas, we need to put the formula into one empty cell. The formula needs to specify the cells which contain the data that you want to calculate the statistic for. All formulas are put in after an ' =' sign.

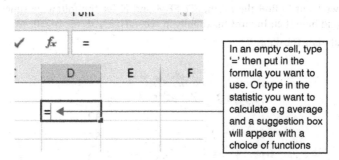

In an empty cell, type '=' then put in the formula you want to use. Or type in the statistic you want to calculate e.g average and a suggestion box will appear with a choice of functions

Once the calculation for that cell is done, then you don't have to repeat typing the formula for the other cells, you can drag the formula across the rows or down the column by highlighting a small black square and dragging this as shown below.

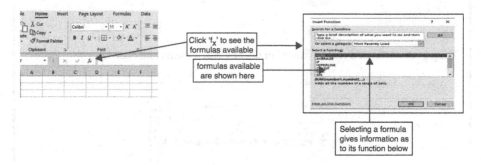

Cell in which the formula is typed. Bring the mouse to the bottom right hand corner of cell- a white cross is seen

Cell in which the formula is typed. Bring the mouse to the bottom right hand corner of cell- the white cross changes to a solid black cross

Click and hold the mouse cursor on the black cross and drag the formula in this cell either downwards or across. The dragged cells will now have the original formula

We can either directly type in the formula as above or use the 'f_x' box just above the columns as shown below.

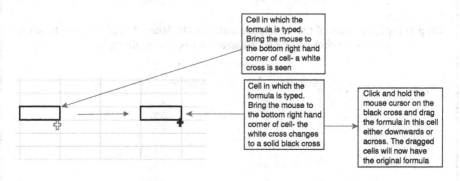

Click 'f_x' to see the formulas available

formulas available are shown here

Selecting a formula gives information as to its function below

EXAMPLE 6.2 | Calculating descriptive statistics using formulas using 'fx'

Suppose we want to find the mean, SD, SEM and N for the following times that six people could hold their breaths maximally in seconds: 37, 55, 63, 24, 50, 42.

Step 1: Tabulate the data

A	B
Subject	**Breathold time (s)**
1	37
2	55
3	63
4	24
5	50
6	42

Step 2: Type the name of the descriptive statistics (N, Mean, SD, SEM) in cells below cell A6. Then click on empty cell adjacent to cell containing N.

A	B
Subject	**Breathold time (s)**
1	37
2	55
3	63
4	24
5	50
6	42
N	
Mean	
SD	
SEM	

Step 3: Click 'fx', and choose 'count' in the box that appears and click OK.

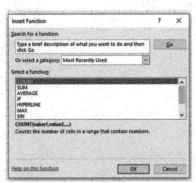

(continued)

EXAMPLE 6.2 *(continued)*

Step 4: In the box that appears, put in the data values (B2:B7) in the Value1 section and click 'OK', the result of **6** will be shown in cell B9.

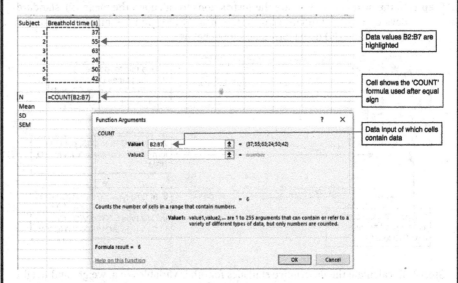

Step 5: Repeat steps 3 and 4 after clicking cell B10 and choosing the function 'Average' and clicking cell B11 and choosing the function 'STDV'. These two functions will calculate mean and standard deviation.

	A	B
1	Subject	Breath hold time (s)
2	1	37
3	2	55
4	3	63
5	4	24
6	5	50
7	6	42
8		
9	N	6
10	Mean	45.2
11	±SD	13.9
12	±SEM	

Step 6: Excel doesn't have a function for SEM. So, to calculate SEM, find the square root of N, and divide this into the SD, i.e.

$$SEM = SD/\sqrt{N}$$

or, $SEM = 13.9/2.4 = 5.79$

Note: We could use the function 'SQRT' to find the square root of N, i.e. =SQRT(6) or above

$= SQRT(B9)$

EXAMPLE 6.3 | Calculating descriptive statistics using formulas typed directly into cells

Step 1: In the boxes (1, 2, 3, 4) are the instructions to calculate the mean ($\bar{x}$), standard deviation (SD), standard error of the mean (SEM) and the number of data for each column (N) using formulae shown below.

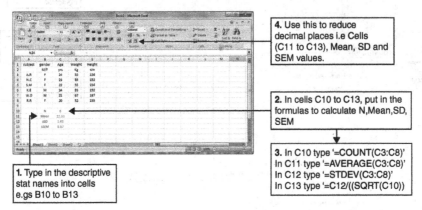

4. Use this to reduce decimal places i.e Cells (C11 to C13), Mean, SD and SEM values.

2. In cells C10 to C13, put in the formulas to calculate N,Mean,SD, SEM

3. In C10 type '=COUNT(C3:C8)'
In C11 type '=AVERAGE(C3:C8)'
In C12 type '=STDEV(C3:C8)'
In C13 type '=C12/((SQRT(C10))

1. Type in the descriptive stat names into cells e.gs B10 to B13

Step 2: To calculate the descriptive statistics for other variables (e.g. weight and height above), there is no need to type in the formulas again. The shortcut is to highlight cell C10, then move the cursor to the extreme right of cell C10, until the black square turns into a black cross, then press down on the left hand mouse button and drag to the right, as you do this the cells D10 and D11 fill with the correct N values. Repeat for the other rows.

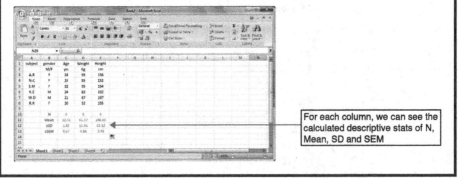

For each column, we can see the calculated descriptive stats of N, Mean, SD and SEM

Using the Data Analysis Tab

An alternative to typing in the formulas (which can be slow and cumbersome) is to use the Data Analysis option in the 'Data' tab. This provides data analysis tools for a wide range of statistical analysis. If you don't see this when you click 'Data' tab, then some additional software (Analysis ToolPak) needs to be set up within Excel.

Setting up the 'Data Analysis' Option on the Toolbar

Step 1: Open Microsoft Excel and click on 'File' from the toolbar (or 'start' on older versions).

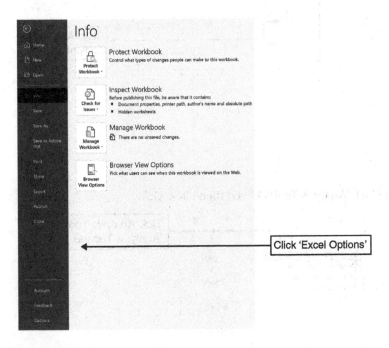

Step 2: Click 'Excel Options'

Step 3: Click 'Add-Ins'.

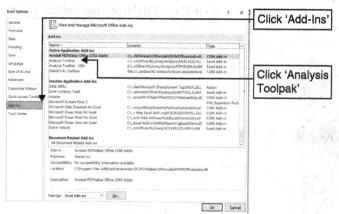

Step 4: Click 'Analysis ToolPak' and then click 'Go'.

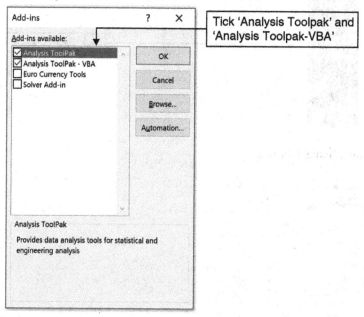

Step 5: A box appears in which you need to tick the 'Analysis ToolPak' and 'Analysis ToolPak VBA' (this will load the software) and then click 'OK'.

Step 6: Click 'Data' on the toolbar (you should now see the 'Data Analysis' option).

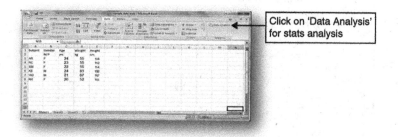

Descriptive Statistics Using the Data Analysis Tab

EXAMPLE 6.4 | Calculating descriptive statistics using data analysis tab

---

Step 1: Click on data tab, then data analysis.

Step 2: Click on descriptive statistics, then OK.

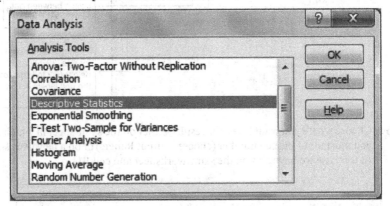

Step 3: Click the option to choose whether your data is in columns or rows, in this example we have chosen columns.

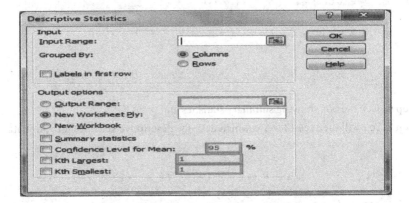

Step 4: In the input range, specify the data for which you want to calculate the descriptive statistics, e.g. in the data above, we want to calculate the descriptive statistics for age (column C), weight (column D) and height (column E). To choose the data click the red arrow in the input box to go to the data, highlight the required data and then click the red arrow again which will return you to the input box

(continued)

EXAMPLE 6.4 *(continued)*

and the data location is now shown in terms of column and row labels. Precaution: check that these labels are correct.

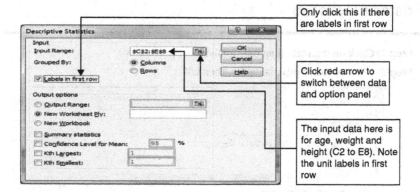

Step 5: Choose where you want to see the results, either on the same sheet in which case you must input the cell number (choose 'Output Range') or on a new worksheet. In this case we have chosen the same worksheet and cell B11.

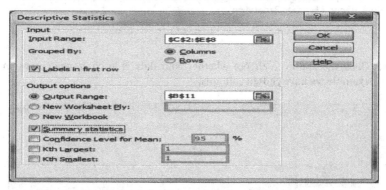

Step 6: Tick the box showing summary statistics and press 'OK'.

Step 7: You will then see 13 terms which describe descriptive statistics for your data.

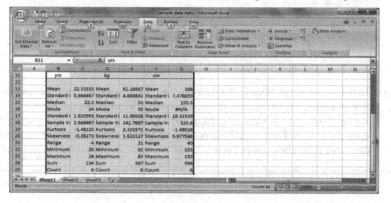

(continued)

EXAMPLE 6.4 *(continued)*

Step 8: Choose the Mean, SD, SEM and count N (and reduce to two decimal places), then put at the end of the columns of data for that variable.

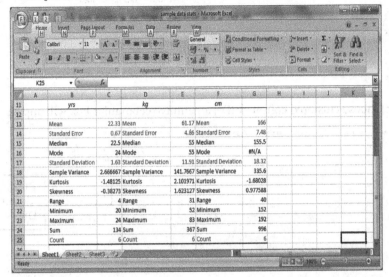

Plotting a Single Bar Graph Using Excel

EXAMPLE 6.5 | Plotting a single bar graph using Excel

Consider the data in Table 6.1 below:

TABLE 6.1 Mean HR and Blood Pressure (±SEM) versus posture

	Control(sitting)			Standing			Supine		
	HR (bmin-)	SP (mmHg)	DP (mmHg)	HR (bmin-)	SP (mmHg)	DP (mmHg)	HR (bmin-)	Sp (mmHg)	DP (mmHg)
MEAN	78.43	115.43	73.71	83.33	115.90	73.52	76.33	119.05	70.52
SEM	2.58	2.50	1.34	2.70	3.33	1.90	2.44	3.15	1.98

Single bar Graphs of Heart Rate Against Posture

Step 1: Open Microsoft Excel and a file showing your data.
Step 2: Click on 'insert', and then click column.

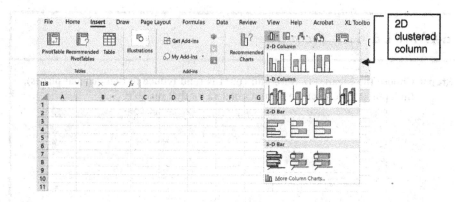

Step 3: Choose clustered column (2D), an empty rectangular box will appear.

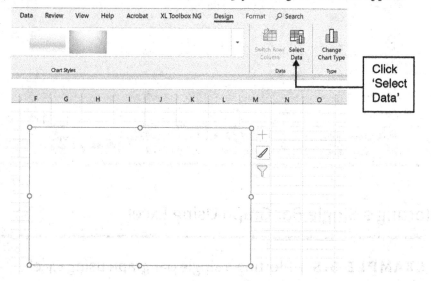

Step 4: Choose 'select data'.
Step 5: Delete anything in the chart data range.

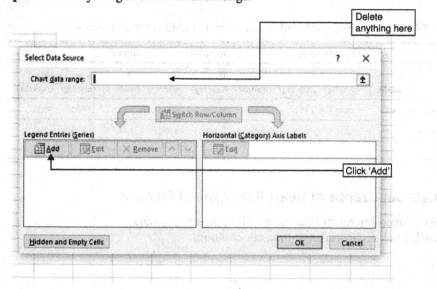

Step 6: Click 'Add' (under legend entries).

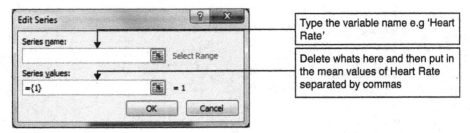

Type the variable name e.g 'Heart Rate'

Delete whats here and then put in the mean values of Heart Rate separated by commas

Step 7: In the series name box, type the variable name, e.g. Heart Rate.

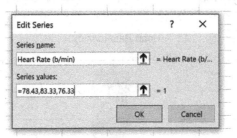

Step 8: In the series values box, type the mean values and click 'OK'.

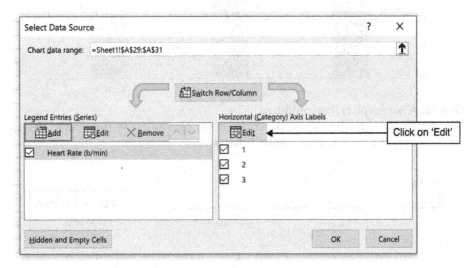

Click on 'Edit'

Step 9: Click 'Edit' in the Horizontal (Category) Axis Labels and type in the labels for each bar, e.g. control, standing, and supine, and then 'OK'.

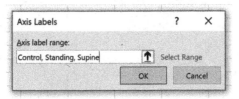

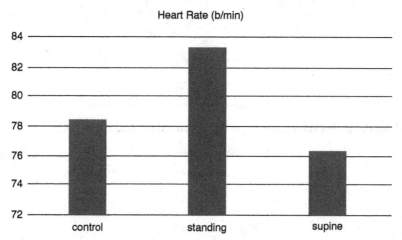

Heart Rate (b/min)

Step 10: A bar graph is then produced.

Step 11: To add error bars (±SEM): click on the rectangle and then click 'Design' from the top row and choose 'Error Bars'.

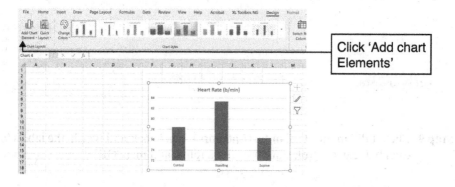

Click 'Add chart Elements'

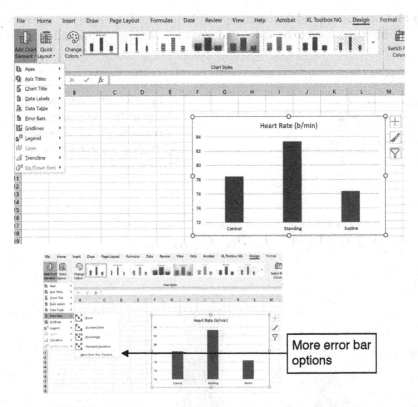

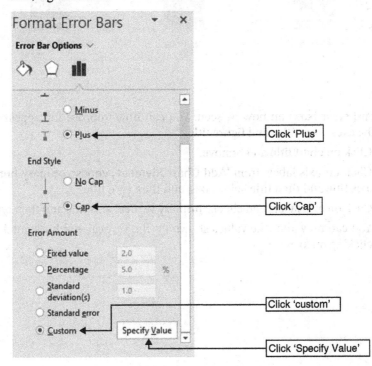

Step 12: Click 'More Error Bar Options' and then choose how to display the error bars, e.g. Plus side.

Step 13: Click custom and then click 'Specify Value', then highlight variable for which error bars need to be added and type in SEM values separated by a comma.

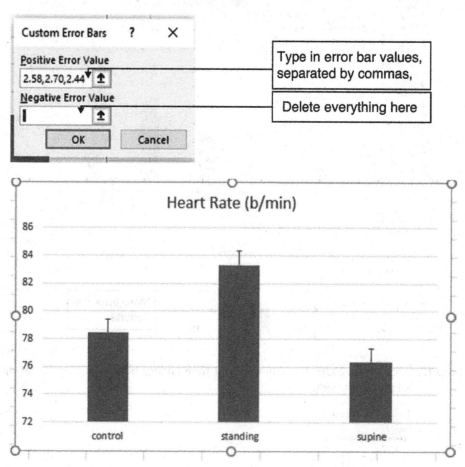

The upward error bars can now be seen. You can now improve the appearance by altering the axes, axes titles and figure title.

Step 14: Click on chart title and remove.

Step 15: Click on axis labels from 'Add Chart Element', choose primary horizontal axis title and then title below axis, and then type title.

Step 16: Click on axis labels and choose primary vertical axis title and then type title.

Step 17: You can now alter the values shown on the vertical and horizontal axis by clicking on axes.

Step 18: Finally add a figure number and title at the bottom below the x axis, by clicking on insert text box and typing the title.

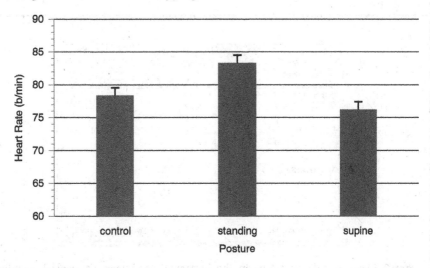

Plotting a Multiple Bar Graph Using Excel

EXAMPLE 6.6 | Multiple bar graphs using Excel

Consider the data shown in Table 6.2.

TABLE 6.2   Mean and SEM blood pressure in different postures

	Control (sitting)		Standing		Supine	
	SP(mmHg)	DP(mmHg)	SP(mmHg)	DP(mmHg)	SP(mmHg)	DP(mmHg)
MEAN	115.43	73.71	115.90	73.52	119.05	70.52
SEM	2.50	1.34	3.33	1.90	3.15	1.98

Step 1: Click insert, then column or bar chart, then 2D clustered Column, select data, then Add and type in Systolic Pressure.

Step 2: To add another bar next to Systolic Pressure, i.e. Diastolic Pressure; click 'Add' and then type 'Diastolic Pressure'.

(continued)

EXAMPLE 6.6 *(continued)*

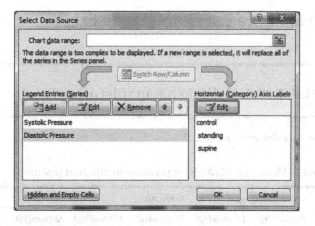

Step 3: Click on 'Edit' and type in the horizontal conditions, i.e. control, standing, and supine.

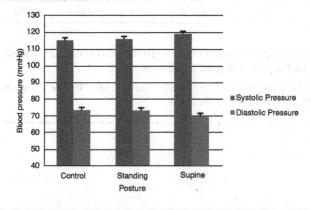

Step 4: A bar graph is then produced.

EXAMPLE 6.6 *(continued)*

Note: to add the error bars, you need to choose 'Add Chart Element', then error bars, then 'more error bar options', then error bar based on series or variable (i.e. systolic and diastolic pressures), then as before choose upward error bars, cap, custom values and then type in the SEM separated by a comma.

Plotting a Stacked Bar Plot Using Excel

EXAMPLE 6.7 | Using a stacked bar to plot a Gantt chart with Microsoft Excel

In a research proposal or project it is common to produce a timeline of tasks in planning the project. Here are the steps in producing the Gantt chart shown in Figure 1.1.

Step 1: In 3 columns put in the tasks, the start date and the end date information.

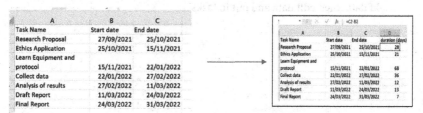

Step 2: Set up an extra column, call it duration in days. Put the following formula in cell D2, ' = C2-B2' and drag this formula to D8, to get duration for each task.

Step 3: Highlight the start dates in column B, then click insert, choose stacked bar from options.

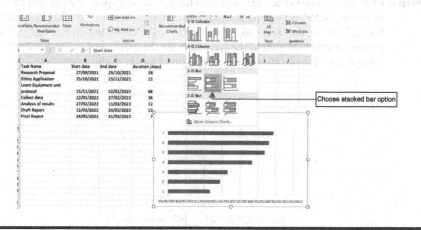

(continued)

EXAMPLE 6.7 (*continued*)

Step 4: Right click on any blue bar, and choose 'select data', put in the duration data.

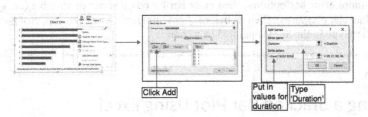

Click Add

Put in values for duration

Type 'Duration'

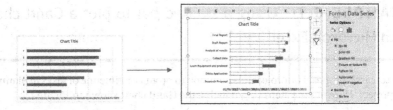

Step 5: Double click on the blue bar and choose 'no fill', then right click on vertical axis, add data, then edit data and put in tasks.

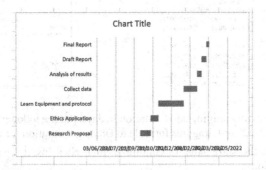

Step 6: Click on tasks on vertical axis and from the format axis option choose 'categories in reverse order'. Next copy the cells containing the start date of the tasks and the end date of the final task to any empty cells. Using the format cell option choose 'General'. Highlight the start dates on the graph, and put in the 2 numbers produced in the minimum and maximum boxes of the axis options.

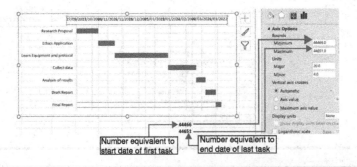

Number equivalent to start date of first task

Number equivalent to end date of last task

Plotting a Scatter Graph with Excel

EXAMPLE 6.8 | Plotting a scatter plot with Microsoft Excel

Suppose you wish to see if there is a relationship between two variables you have measured (e.g. lung size and height of subject, absorbance and concentration, applied force and extension of material) then you can do a scatter plot and calculate the correlation coefficient (r^2).

Table 6.3 shows the absorbance data obtained from a spectrophotometer for a series of concentrations of copper sulphate

TABLE 6.3 Absorbances of copper sulphate concentrations

Concentration of copper sulphate (mg L^{-1})	0	0.50	0.75	1.00	1.25	1.50	1.75	2.00
Absorbance	0	0.121	0.192	0.251	0.345	0.380	0.453	0.510

Step 1: Put the above data into two columns and highlight all including column names.

(continued)

EXAMPLE 6.8 *(continued)*

Step 2: Click 'Insert' and then from the chart's choices click on scatter X,Y charts. The following chart will be produced.

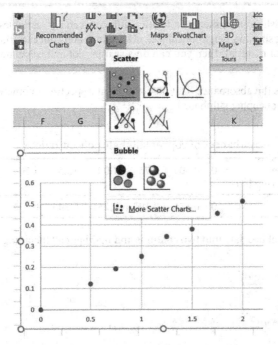

Step 3: Click on the chart and the 'Design' tab options are highlighted.

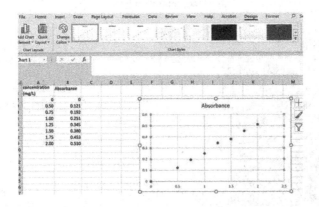

Note: if you want to swap the order of the Y and X axis values, then you need to choose 'select data' either by right clicking on the chart (or from the Design tab) and using the 'edit' option to change the values for the X and Y series.

(continued)

EXAMPLE 6.8 *(continued)*

Step 4: Within the 'Design tab' you will see two options called 'Quick Layout' and 'Add Chart Element'. The 'Quick Layout' tab gives 11 layout options for your scatter plot (choose one of these). Now click 'Add Chart Element' and various optional features can be added to the plot (e.g. axis labels, title, error bars, trendline, etc). Choose 'trendline' and then click on 'linear'. A straight line plot is then produced. Now click on 'More Trendline Options' from the trendline choices or double click on the 'Straight line' and a 'Format Trendline' box will appear.

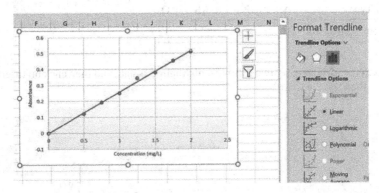

Step 5: Scroll down on 'Format Trendline' and then tick the boxes for 'Display Equation' and 'R-squared'.

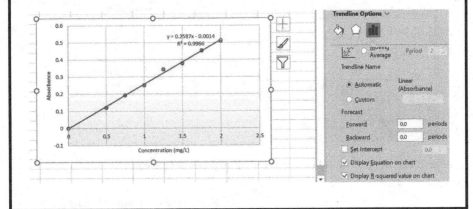

The above linear plot is shown with the equation for the straight line and the R-squared value (R^2) showing the correlation.

Plotting a Pie Chart Using Excel

EXAMPLE 6.9 | Plotting a pie chart using Microsoft Excel

Consider the data of blood types obtained from a cohort of students below in Table 6.4.

TABLE 6.4	Blood types of a student cohort			
Blood Type	A	B	AB	O
Number of students	10	8	5	12

Step 1: Type in data under two columns, highlight this data and then click on Insert and then '2D Pie Chart'.

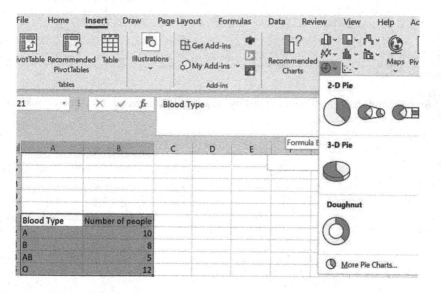

Step 2: Use 'design' and 'add chart elements' to produce final chart.

Plotting a Frequency Distribution Graph Using Excel

EXAMPLE 6.10 | Plotting a frequency distribution curve with Excel

Using the data in Example 2.4 from Chapter 2.

The number of red blood cells in millions/microlitre, measured from 15 students, is shown below:

3.5, 6.9, 5.5, 6.0, 4.3, 5.1, 4.7, 6.3, 5.2, 6.3, 5.9, 5.7, 5.8, 5.2, 6.1

Step 1: Set up a data table into Excel showing class widths and frequency.

Class width	Frequency
3.5 <4.0	1
4.0 <4.5	1
4.5<5.0	1
5.0<5.5	3
5.5<6.0	4
6.0<6.5	4
6.5<7.0	1

(Ctrl) ▾

Step 2: Highlight the above two columns, click Insert and click on column chart or recommended chart.

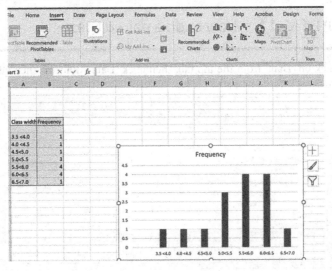

(continued)

EXAMPLE 6.10 *(continued)*

Step 3: Fine tune the graph with appropriate labels.

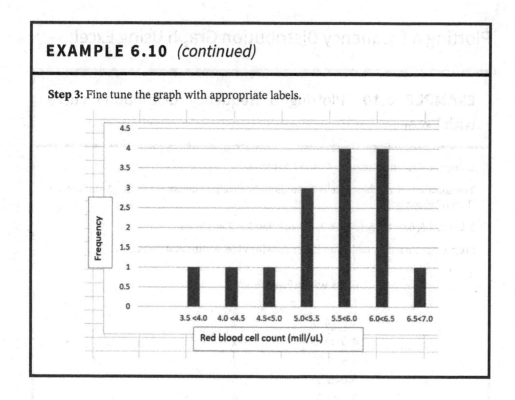

Inferential Statistics with Microsoft Excel

Paired t-test with Excel

EXAMPLE 6.11 | How to do a paired t-test

Step 1: Click on 'Data' from the top tab, then click 'Data Analysis', then click 't-Test: Paired Two Sample for Means', then 'OK'.

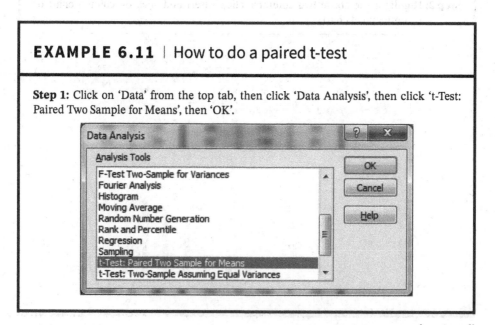

(continued)

EXAMPLE 6.11 *(continued)*

Step 2: For 'Variable 1 Range' = put in the cell numbers which contain the data (alternatively, click on the red arrow and highlight the data and click red arrow again).

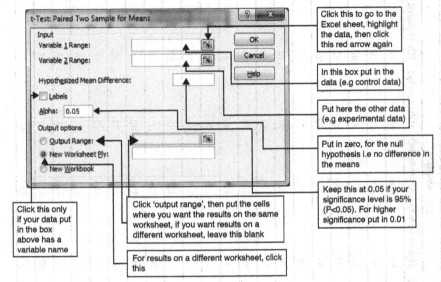

Step 3: For 'Variable 2 Range' = put in the cell numbers which contain the data (alternatively, click on the red arrow and highlight the data and click red arrow again).

Step 4: For 'Hypothesized Mean Difference' = put zero.

Step 5: Choose where the output of the analysis should be shown (same sheet, new sheet, or new workbook), click 'OK'.

Step 6: A two column table will appear which is interpreted for significance as follows:

i. if the T value is greater than the '2 tail predicted T value' the difference in the means is significant

ii. if the 'P' value is less than the predicted 2 tail P value of 0.05, then the result is significant.

Example of a Paired t-test

The table below (Table 6.5) shows the changes in blood pressure and heart rate in different postures. Suppose you want to know whether there is a significant difference in the mean systolic pressure between control and standing postures. We will now follow steps 1–6 from example 6.11 above.

TABLE 6.5 Blood pressure and heart rate versus posture

	A	B	C	D	E	F	G	H	I	J	K	L	M	N
10			Age	Weight	Height	Control(sitting)			Standing			supine		
ii	Subject	M/F	yrs	Kg	cm	HR (bmin-1)	SP(mmHg)	DP(mmHg)	HR (bmin-1)	SP(mmHg)	DP(mmHg)	HR (bmin-1)	SP(mmHg)	DP(mmHg)
12	K.B	F	20	50	160	91	117	80	96	103	69	79	112	66
13	R.R	F	19	50	156	91	120	80	98	100	70	80	120	60
14	L.M	M	28	67	181	65	108	73	83	107	74	62	106	61
15	S.S	M	21	76	175	81	138	79	92	145	84	82	143	76
16	K.E	M	24	84	189	86	110	70	99	107	75	80	128	73
17	M.S	M	24	97	183	71	119	71	80	112	72	67	124	65
la	S.R	F	19	55	168	60	97	73	70	82	54	72	93	58
15	A.J	M	20	71	167	74	119	68	79	125	67	67	130	69
zo	M.S	M	21	84	190	77	117	75	89	106	75	80	119	66
21	Y.O	F	21	65	164	86	129	73	91	124	83	94	125	75
22	AR	F	21	52	165	79	126	68	88	135	76	87	123	70
23	SV	F	28	60	168	84	118	72	90	111	69	78	101	62
24	SR	F	22	57	161.5	90	112	85	81	138	89	87	121	80
26	CC	F	19	48	164	67	104	72	76	110	80	75	104	70
26	O.F	M	24	75	175	62	126	65	66	129	62	67	122	65
27	T.S	F	21	62	150	89	100	76	95	108	74	90	109	66
za	DG	F	22	55	159	92	116	73	91	108	72	87	112	69
zo	DR	F	23	75	172	82	99	70	91	111	71	80	121	81
30	FS	M	28	71	182	79	117	61	62	126	84	53	135	82
31	SH	F	30	82	163	90	99	78	80	110	60	82	100	70
32	PB	M	45	98	189	51	133	86	53	137	84	54	152	97
33														

Put in the control data (sitting) for systolic pressures into the 'Variable 1 Range' box. Put in the standing data for systolic pressures into the 'Variable 2 Range' box.

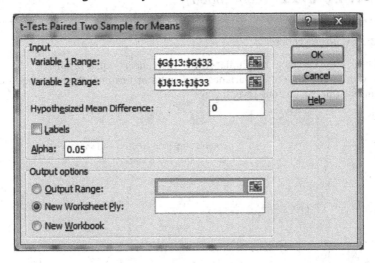

The following results are shown:

t-Test: Paired Two Sample for Means

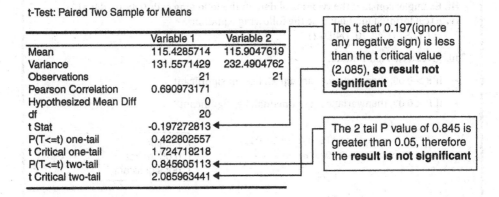

	Variable 1	Variable 2
Mean	115.4285714	115.9047619
Variance	131.5571429	232.4904762
Observations	21	21
Pearson Correlation	0.690973171	
Hypothesized Mean Diff	0	
df	20	
t Stat	-0.197272813	
P(T<=t) one-tail	0.422802557	
t Critical one-tail	1.724718218	
P(T<=t) two-tail	0.845605113	
t Critical two-tail	2.085963441	

The 't stat' 0.197(ignore any negative sign) is less than the t critical value (2.085), **so result not significant**

The 2 tail P value of 0.845 is greater than 0.05, therefore the **result is not significant**

Independent t-tests

EXAMPLE 6.12 | How to do an unpaired (independent) t-test and F-test

Firstly, note that the sample sizes in your two independent groups are different.

Step 1: Click 'Data', then 'Data Analysis', then you see two options, (i) two samples with equal variances, or (ii) two samples with unequal variances.

(continued)

EXAMPLE 6.12 *(continued)*

Step 2: How do you choose?

i.   Check if the variances are similar- if yes- then choose equal variances.
ii. If you are not sure if the variances are equal or unequal, then use the F-test to check—this can be done several ways.

	A	B	C	D	E	F
1						
2			Sleep duration in controls and snorers			
3			control (hr)	snorers(hr)		
4			6	4		
5			8	6		
6			6.5	5		
7			9	4.5		
8			5	4		
9			7	5.5		
10			8	3		
11				5		
12				4		

iii. Example: consider the two sets of data in the following cells (c4:c10; d4: d12)
iv. Excel formula method: type the following equation:
= FTEST (C4:C10, D4:D12)

This gives a two tail P value.

*   if $P > 0.05$, then variances are equal, i.e. not significant

*   if $P < 0.05$, then variances are unequal, i.e. significant

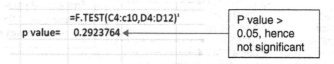

	=F.TEST(C4:c10,D4:D12)'
p value=	0.2923764

P value > 0.05, hence not significant

v. Data Analysis tab method: choose F-test, then put in the two groups of data and click 'OK'.

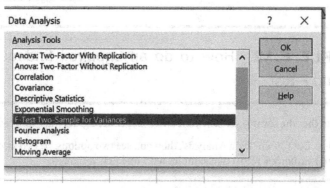

(continued)

EXAMPLE 6.12 (*continued*)

F-Test Two-Sample for Variances   ?   ✕

Input
Variable <u>1</u> Range: $C$3:$C$10   ⬆   OK
Variable <u>2</u> Range: $D$3:$D$12   ⬆   Cancel

☑ <u>L</u>abels   <u>H</u>elp
<u>A</u>lpha: 0.05

Output options
◉ <u>O</u>utput Range: $G$3   ⬆
◯ New Worksheet <u>P</u>ly:
◯ New <u>W</u>orkbook

F-Test Two-Sample for Variances

	control (hr)	snorers(hr)
Mean	7.07142857	4.555555556
Variance	1.86904762	0.840277778
Observations	7	9
df	6	8
F	2.22432113	
P(F<=f) one-tail	0.14618819 ◀	
F Critical one-tail	3.58058032 ◀	

Since F is less than Fcritical, not significant, variances are equal

Multiply this by 2 to obtain 2 tail P value, the answer is > 0.05, hence not significant

vi. Equation method: F value = larger variance/smaller variance.
Or F = 1.869 047 62/0.840 277 778

$$= 2.224\ 321\ 134$$

Compare this with the $F_{critical}$ value (obtained from F table using df for larger variance (6) and df for smaller variance (8), i.e. $F_{critical} = 3.58$.

Since $F_{value} < F_{critical}$, then the result is not significant, and variances are equal.

Step 3: Carry out the relevant unpaired t-test (i.e. two sample with equal variance).

t-Test: Two-Sample Assuming Equal Variances   ?   ✕

Input
Variable <u>1</u> Range: $C$3:$C$10   ⬆   OK
Variable <u>2</u> Range: $D$3:$D$12   ⬆   Cancel

Hypoth<u>e</u>sized Mean Difference: 0   <u>H</u>elp

☑ <u>L</u>abels
<u>A</u>lpha: 0.05

Output options
◉ <u>O</u>utput Range: $M$5   ⬆
◯ New Worksheet <u>P</u>ly:
◯ New <u>W</u>orkbook

(*continued*)

EXAMPLE 6.12 (continued)

Step 4: See if there is significance.

t-Test: Two-Sample Assuming Equal Variances

	control (hr)	snorers(hr)
Mean	7.07142857	4.5555556
Variance	1.86904762	0.8402778
Observations	7	9
Pooled Variance	1.28117914	
Hypothesized Mean Difference	0	
df	14	
t Stat	4.41056342	
P(T<=t) one-tail	0.00029632	
t Critical one-tail	1.76131014	
P(T<=t) two-tail	0.00059265	
t Critical two-tail	2.14478669	

A significant result

One-way ANOVA with Excel

EXAMPLE 6.13 | How to do one-way ANOVA

FEV_1 was measured in three groups (each group had three people) as shown in Table 6.6.

TABLE 6.6 Changes of FEV_1 in healthy, smoking, and obese groups

Groups	Control	Smokers	Obese
FEV_1 Values (L)	3.90	2.65	3.10
	3.65	2.40	3.35
	4.0	2.20	3.80

Step 1: From the Data Analysis tab, choose 'Anova Single Factor', click 'OK'.

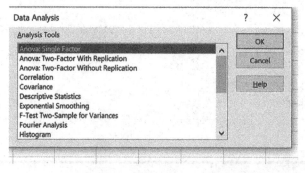

EXAMPLE 6.13 *(continued)*

Step 2: Put in the input range the three groups of data, click labels, set alpha as 0.05, set output range, click 'OK'.

Anova: Single Factor ? ×

Input

Input Range: $C$5:$E$8

Grouped By: ◉ Columns
○ Rows

☑ Labels in first row

Alpha: 0.05

Output options

◉ Output Range: $N$4
○ New Worksheet Ply:
○ New Workbook

OK

Cancel

Help

Step 3: If P < 0.05, then there is a significant difference between groups. This is also shown by F value > F critical value.

Anova: Single Factor

SUMMARY

Groups	Count	Sum	Average	Variance
Control	3	11.55	3.85	0.0325
smokers	3	7.25	2.416667	0.050833
obese	3	10.25	3.416667	0.125833

ANOVA

Source of Variation	SS	df	MS	F	P-value	F crit
Between Groups	3.242222	2	1.621111	23.251	0.001493	5.143253
Within Groups	0.418333	6	0.069722			
Total	3.660556	8				

Step 4: If there is no significant difference, then there is no difference in the means between the groups, however, if there is a significant difference, then we need to look at each pair comparisons (i.e. control versus smokers, control versus obese, and smokers versus obese) to see which pairs are significant.

Step 5: To see which pairs are significantly different we have to do post hoc tests. Examples of these are (i) Bonferroni, (ii) Tukey HSD, (iii) Dunnett's, (iv) Fischer's LSD, and (v) Kruseman Kallis.

Post hoc tests

Bonferroni test

EXAMPLE 6.14 | Bonferroni post hoc test

This is a series of t-tests to find the confidence interval for pairs of means. They are follow up tests after ANOVA and are used to find which pairs of means are significant. Each Bonferroni comparison is a confidence interval (CI). If zero is found in the CI, then the null hypothesis is zero, i.e. true or no difference. If zero is not found in the CI, then the null hypothesis is not true and there is a difference in the means, i.e. significant.

Step 1: Do an appropriate t-test for each pair.

t-Test: Paired Two Sample for Means

	Control	smokers
Mean	3.85	2.4166667
Variance	0.0325	0.0508333
Observations	3	3
Pearson Correlatio	-0.21527425	
Hypothesized Mea	0	
df	2	
t Stat	7.818181818	
P(T<=t) one-tail	0.007984677	
t Critical one-tail	2.91998558	
P(T<=t) two-tail	0.015969354	
t Critical two-tail	4.30265273	

t-Test: Paired Two Sample for Means

	Control	obese
Mean	3.85	3.416666667
Variance	0.0325	0.125833333
Observatio	3	3
Pearson C	0.430024	
Hypothesi	0	
df	2	
t Stat	2.334869	
P(T<=t) on	0.072331	
t Critical o	2.919986	
P(T<=t) tw	0.144663	
t Critical t	4.302653	

t-Test: Paired Two Sample for Means

	smokers	obese
Mean	2.416667	3.416666667
Variance	0.050833	0.125833333
Observatio	3	3
Pearson C	-0.97422	
Hypothesi	0	
df	2	
t Stat	-3.00376	
P(T<=t) on	0.04763	
t Critical o	2.919986	
P(T<=t) tw	0.09526	
t Critical t	4.302653	

Step 2: Calculate a new P value threshold as follows:

New P value = old P value /number of comparisons

    For this example, old P value = 0.05; number of comparisons = 3

    Thus, new P value = 0.05/3 = 0.0167.

Step 3: Check if the above p values (two tail) are < 0.0167, which would then show significance.

From the above, we can see that all three pairs of comparisons show a significant difference.

Tukey HSD Post Hoc Test

This compares sample means using their absolute differences.

Step 1: Calculate the Tukey criterion (T) using the formula below:

$$T = q_{\alpha (c, N-C)} \sqrt{(MSE/n_i)}$$

Where,

$\alpha = 0.05$, C = number of treatments or groups; N = total sample size; MSE = mean square error (within groups), n_i = sample size of the treatment group with the smallest number of observations, q = critical value based on number of groups and degrees of freedom = (N-C).

Step 2: For this example, C = 3, N = 9, thus df = 9-3 = 6, q = x (from tables).
Step 3: Calculate the absolute mean differences for each pair:
control versus smokers = 3.85–2.416
control versus obese = 3.85–3.416
smokers versus obese = 2.416–3.416.
Step 4: If the absolute value is > T, then it is significant; if less, then it is not significant.

Two-way ANOVA using Excel

EXAMPLE 6.15 | How to do two-way ANOVA

Table 6.7 shows the reaction times in msec measured on three devices (ruler, computer, and light device) by three males (M) and three females (F).

TABLE 6.7 Effect of gender and reaction time devices on reaction time (ms)

Gender	Reaction Time Device		
	Ruler	computer	light device
M1	300	230	240
M2	350	210	250
M2	400	200	300
F1	280	250	260
F2	350	315	300
F3	400	320	315

From this data we are asking the two major questions:

i) is there a difference in the reaction times between genders?
ii) is there a difference in reaction times between the three devices?

A third possible question would be is there any interactions or influence which may affect the performance between genders and the use of the reaction time devices (e.g. could they have used these devices before).

There are two main factors here, one is gender and the other is type of device. So, we will use two-way ANOVA. Excel allows you to choose with replication and without replication. With replication involves studies with different subjects and experiments and is more common. Without replication tends to have only a single measurement for each factor.

For this example, the ANOVA with replication is the one to choose.

(continued)

EXAMPLE 6.15 (continued)

Step 1: Set up a data table as above, then click the Data tab, then Data analysis and choose 'ANOVA Two-Factor With Replication' and click 'OK'.

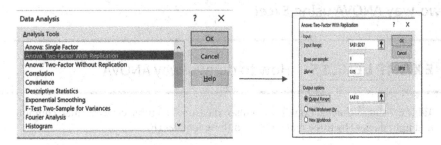

Step 2: Highlight all the data for the table and put in the input range, as there are three males and three females, put three in the sample and after selecting output range click 'OK'.

Anova: Two-Factor With Replication

SUMMARY	Ruler	computer	light device	Total
M1				
Count	3	3	3	9
Sum	1050	640	790	2480
Average	350	213.3333	263.3333	275.5556
Variance	2500	233.3333	1033.333	4527.778
F1				
Count	3	3	3	9
Sum	1030	885	875	2790
Average	343.3333	295	291.6667	310
Variance	3633.333	1525	808.3333	2118.75
Total				
Count	6	6	6	
Sum	2080	1525	1665	
Average	346.6667	254.1667	277.5	
Variance	2466.667	2704.167	977.5	

ANOVA						
Source of Varia	SS	df	MS	F	P-value	F crit
Sample	5338.889	1	5338.889	3.291096	0.094721	4.747225
Columns	27769.44	2	13884.72	8.559075	0.004899	3.885294
Interaction	5936.111	2	2968.056	1.829623	0.202517	3.885294
Within	19466.67	12	1622.222			
Total	58511.11	17				

As F value is < Forit and the P value is >0.05, the effect of gender is not significant

As F> Forit and P< 0.05, there is a significant difference between the devices

Interaction not significant (F< Forit; P>0.05)

Step 3: The sample is the rows (gender) and the columns is the devices. Only the devices show a significant difference and a post hoc test would need to be done to see which devices are showing a significant effect. The interaction between gender and devices is not significant and thus one doesn't affect the other.

Summary

- Microsoft Excel is an electronic spreadsheet which stores, organizes, calculates, and displays data. It is organized in rows and columns.
- This software communicates easily with other software such as GraphPad Prism and SPSS for importing and exporting data.
- Statistical analysis of data can be performed with formula functions and by using the 'Data Analysis' tab under the 'Data' tab to calculate descriptive and inferential tests.
- Data can be displayed in tables or in graphs. The 'Insert' tab and then 'chart function' can be used to draw various types of graphs (e.g. bar charts, frequency distribution, scatter, and line graphs) together with error bars.
- Examples of inferential tests (e.g. parametric tests, t-tests, correlations, ANOVA) are shown including how to test for significance.
- Non-parametric tests are not available on Excel, however, macros and formulas can be used to do these.

CHAPTER 7

Using Prism
Descriptive and Inferential Statistics

Expected Learning Outcomes

- Describe the structure and layout of Prism.
- Input data into Prism.
- Calculate descriptive statistics using Prism.
- Analyse and interpret inferential statistics using Prism.

What is Graphpad Prism

Prism is a statistical software package which is used widely in science, particularly in biosciences. In the author's opinion, this package is excellent for drawing graphs because of the ease of altering and fine tuning the graphs and the help menus are very good. The statistical analysis is also more than adequate for most studies. Please see Appendix 6 about familiarization with Prism (structure and layout) and the different versions of Prism. Higher versions of Prism can be downloaded for free from the websites for 30-day use, these have more detail on statistics, but the earlier versions are more than enough for most graphs and statistical analysis. The details below are based on using Prism 4 or below. Please note that data created in higher versions cannot be manipulated in lower versions.

Start Prism

To start Prism, double click on the GraphPad Prism software and a welcome to Graphpad Prism template will open as shown below.

Essential Statistics for Bioscientists, First Edition. Mohammed Meah.
© 2022 John Wiley & Sons Ltd. Published 2022 by John Wiley & Sons Ltd.

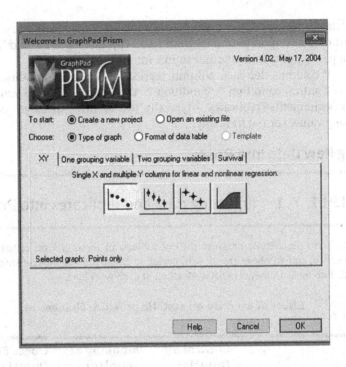

Inputting Data into Prism

Click 'OK', this exits the Welcome template and shows an empty data table. There are five tabs at the top (Data, Results, Graphs, Layout, Notes) and on the side. Of these Data, Results and Graphs are the most important. The other three tabs that are important are 'New', 'Analyze' and 'Change'.

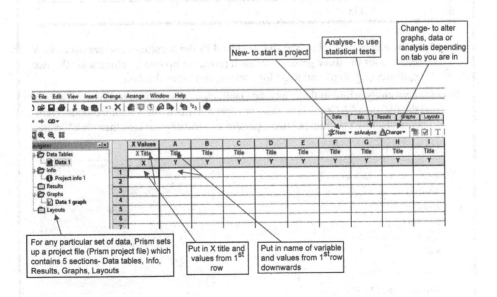

With the Data tab open, and the cursor placed on row 1 of the X column, you can now type in your data or import your data from Excel (by clicking 'File' and 'Import') or cutting and pasting data from another source into the table.

For the Y columns, let each column represent a different condition for each variable, i.e. Control, condition 1, condition 2. Under each of these you could put repeated measurements (replicates – typically two or three usually – don't worry about missing values) or not have any.

Inputting Raw Data Into Prism

EXAMPLE 7.1 | Inputting data and replicates into Prism

Table 7.1 shows the systolic pressure (SP) of subjects in three groups: control group, smoking group, and an obese group, who cycled to exhaustion against an incremental workload. Two measurements of SP were taken at each workload.

TABLE 7.1	Effect of exercise on systolic pressure changes in three groups					
		Control SP (mmHg)		Smoking SP (mmHg)		Obese SP (mmHg)	
Subject	Workload (W)	Rep 1	Rep 2	Rep 1	Rep 2	Rep 1	Rep 2
1	0						
2	50						
3	100						
4	125						
5	150						
6	175						

Step 1: In the empty data table, put the workload in the X column and set up three Y columns for the three groups. For each group set up two Y columns for the two replicates (e.g. Rep1 and Rep2 for control) and input the data.

Step 2: Alternatively, whilst in the empty data table, click 'New' tab, then choose 'New Data Table (+Graph)'. A Create New Table box opens. In this in the X column, choose Numbers and under Y column put two replicates to calculate error bars, then click 'Create'.

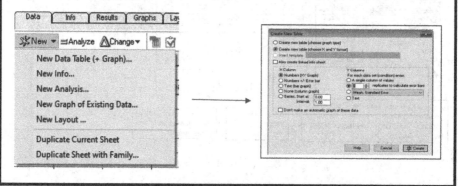

(continued)

EXAMPLE 7.1 (continued)

Step 3: The following format table is produced, now change the titles and put in your data.

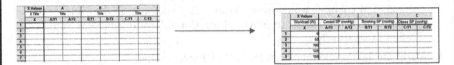

The replicates will be used by Prism to calculate the means and SEM (or SD depending on your choice). If you already have the mean data and error bars calculated, then you can still plot the graphs (see example 7.2 below).

Inputting Mean Data Into Prism

EXAMPLE 7.2 | Inputting calculated means, SEMs or SD data into Prism

Step 1: If you have calculated the descriptive statistics (example in Excel) and you want to plot them in Prism, first display it in a table, see Table 7.2.

TABLE 7.2 Mean blood pressure, heart rate and SEM during control and exercise

	Blood Pressure (mmHg)		Heart Rate	
	SP (mmHg)	SEM	b/min	SEM
Control	130	5.5	75	5
Exercise	165	8.4	160	10

Step 2: (i) Start with 'Data' tab open, then click 'New DataTable (+Graph)', a box will appear called Create New Table, (ii) click 'work independently', (iii) set X column to 'Text', (iv) set Y column to 'Mean, Standard Error'

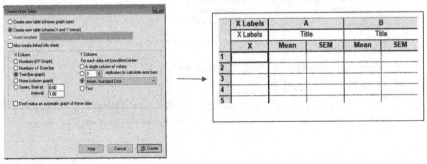

(continued)

Step 3: Click 'Create new table (choose X and Y format)', set X Column to 'Text (bar graph)'and Y Column to 'Mean,Standard Error' and then click 'Create'.

Step 4: The empty data table is now set up, In the 'X Labels' column, row 1 and 2 would have 'Control' and 'Exercise' respectively. In the 'A' column, the 'Title' would be replaced with the variable name 'SP (mmHg) and for 'Control' label the mean and SEM columns would have 130 and 5.5. In column 'B' the 'Title' would be replaced by 'Heart Rate (b/min) and the 'Control' mean and SEM would be 75 and 5 respectively.

Similarly, the data would then be put in for the 'Exercise' label.

Graphical Display   Once you have put data in the data table, an initial graphical display of the data can be seen by clicking 'Graphs' tab on the left side of the page.

You can customize the graph using the 'Change' tab at the top of the screen and choosing various sub-menus. However, the simplest and most common is to click or double click on the parts of the graph you want to alter (e.g. axes, symbols, legends and titles). The flexibility to fine tune graphs in Prism is excellent.

Statistical Analysis

When you are in the 'Data' tab, click the 'Analyze' button.

An Analyze Data box will appear, then choosing Statistical analysis gives various statistical choices and choosing Curves & Regression allows you to fit a curve or do regression.

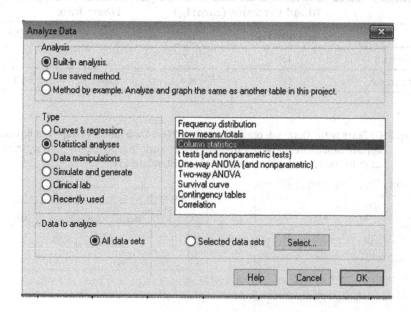

Descriptive Statistics

EXAMPLE 7.3 | Calculating the mean, SD, and SEM in Prism

Human placental lactogen (HPL) hormone was measured in 25 women between 36 and 39 weeks of pregnancy (Table 7.3).

TABLE 7.3 | **HPL levels in women**

Subject	1	2	3	4	5	6	7	8	9	10	11	12	13	14	15	16	17	18	19	20	21	22	23	24	25
HPL (mg/L)	6.1	7.9	6.6	13.1	5.8	4.8	7.4	7.9	10.9	5.8	5.2	9.2	5.5	5.0	8.9	5.8	6.9	5.5	7.5	7.1	12.2	9.9	6.1	7.0	11.3

Step 1: In column A, delete title and replace with the variable name HPL, then put data in the rows.

Step 2: Click 'Analyze', then choose 'Statistical analysis' and 'Column statistics' and click 'OK'.

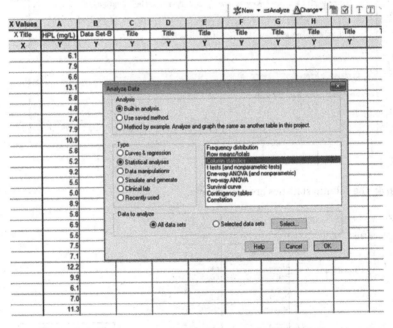

Step 3: In the next box, tick the boxes for the Descriptive Statistic parameters you require and click 'OK'. In this case we need mean, standard deviation, and standard error, but I have ticked other parameters as well.

(continued)

EXAMPLE 7.3 (continued)

Parameters: Column Statistics

Descriptive Statistics
- ☑ Minimum and maximum
- ☑ Quartiles (Median, 25th and 75th percentile)
- ☑ Mean, SD, SEM
- ☑ 95% CI of the mean
- ☐ Coefficient of variation
- ☐ Geometric mean with 95% CI
- ☐ Skewness and kurtosis

Test if the values come from a Gaussian distribution
- ☐ Kolmogorov-Smirnov test (with Dallal-Wilkinson-Lilliefor P value)
- ☐ D'Agostino and Pearson omnibus normality test (recommended)
- ☐ Shapiro-Wilk normality test

Inferences
- ☐ One-sample t test. Are column means significantly different than a hypothetical value?
- ☐ Wilcoxon signed-rank test. Compare column medians to a hypothetical value?

Hypothetical value (often 0.0, 1.0 or 100) | 0.0000

Options
Confidence Intervals: ○ 90% ● 95% ○ 99% ○ ☐ %
Show 4 ⌄ significant digits

[Help Me Decide]   [Cancel]   [OK]

Step 4: The column statistics are now shown.

or			A
Data Tables			HPL
Data 1			Y
Info	1	Number of values	25
Project info 1	2		
Results	3	Minimum	4.800
Col Stats of Data 1	4	25% Percentile	5.800
Graphs	5	Median	7.000
Data 1 graph	6	75% Percentile	9.050
Layouts	7	Maximum	13.10
	8		
	9	Mean	7.576 ◄
	10	Std. Deviation	2.338 ◄
	11	Std. Error	0.4677 ◄
	12		
	13	Lower 95% CI of mean	6.611
	14	Upper 95% CI of mean	8.541
	15		
	16	Sum	189.4
	17		
	18		
	19		
	20		

The mean and standard deviation and standard error are shown here

Plotting a Histogram

EXAMPLE 7.4 | Plotting a histogram in Prism

We will use the data from example 7.1.

Step 1: Click 'New' then choose 'New Analysis'.

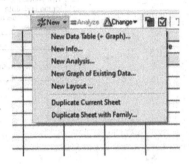

Step 2: Then choose Statistical analysis and Frequency distribution and click 'Create'.

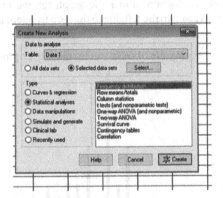

Step 3: Since the data does not have frequency already calculated, Prism will calculate the frequencies. To do this it will automatically decide on the number of classes (or bins), the bin width and the centre of the bin, if the 'Automatic bins' is ticked as shown below and click 'OK'.

Choosing automatic bins, for this data, will mean the bin width is 0.5 and the centre of the first bin is 0.0

(continued)

EXAMPLE 7.4 (continued)

Step 4: This produces the histogram data for plotting the graph.

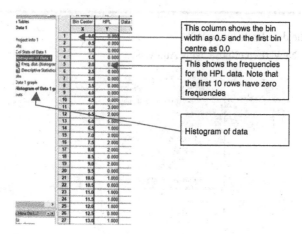

This column shows the bin width as 0.5 and the first bin centre as 0.0

This shows the frequencies for the HPL data. Note that the first 10 rows have zero frequencies

Histogram of data

Step 5: If we now click 'Histogram' under the graph tab we produce the histogram below, which is skewed to the left due to the zero frequencies in the first 10 rows.

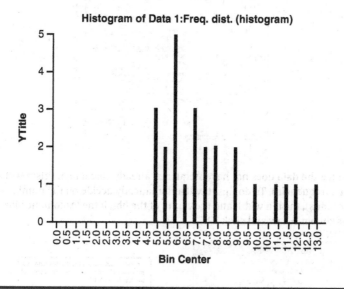

Histogram of Data 1:Freq. dist. (histogram)

(continued)

EXAMPLE 7.4 *(continued)*

Step 6: To improve this click 'Change' and choose 'Analysis Parameters'.

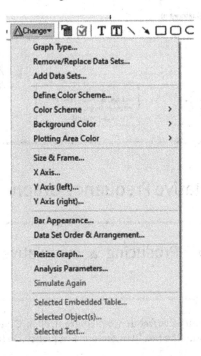

Step 7: This will give the frequency distribution parameter box. Uncheck 'Automatic bins' and put in a bin width of 1.0 and make the centre of the bin as 5.0. and click 'OK'.

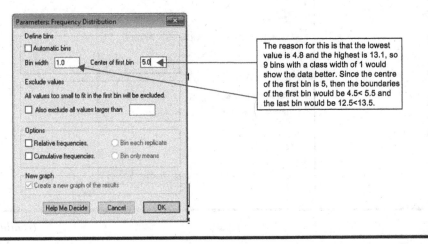

The reason for this is that the lowest value is 4.8 and the highest is 13.1, so 9 bins with a class width of 1 would show the data better. Since the centre of the first bin is 5, then the boundaries of the first bin would be 4.5< 5.5 and the last bin would be 12.5<13.5.

(continued)

EXAMPLE 7.4 (*continued*)

Step 8: This now produces a better histogram.

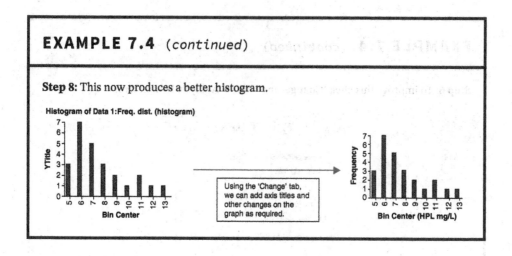

Histogram of Data 1:Freq. dist. (histogram)

Using the 'Change' tab, we can add axis titles and other changes on the graph as required.

Plotting a Cumulative Frequency Graph

EXAMPLE 7.5 | Producing a cumulative frequency plot using Prism

Step 1: To produce a cumulative frequency histogram, click 'Change' and choose 'Analysis parameters' and the box 'Parameters: Frequency Distribution' is shown.

Parameters: Frequency Distribution

Define bins
☐ Automatic bins
Bin width 1.0   Center of first bin 5.0

Exclude values
All values too small to fit in the first bin will be excluded.
☐ Also exclude all values larger than

Options
☐ Relative frequencies.   ◯ Bin each replicate
☑ Cumulative frequencies.   ◯ Bin only means

New graph
☑ Create a new graph of the results

Help Me Decide   Cancel   OK

(*continued*)

EXAMPLE 7.5 *(continued)*

Step 2: Tick 'Cumulative frequencies' and 'OK' and the cumulative frequencies and bin centres are shown, from which the cumulative frequency histogram can be seen below.

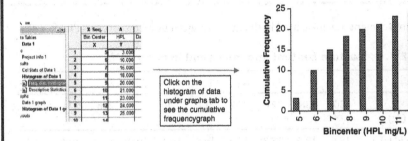

Click on the histogram of data under graphs tab to see the cumulative frequencygraph

Step 3: To obtain the median and interquartile range (which have already been given under the Descriptive Statistics results) from the cumulative frequency graph, it would be easier to change the cumulative frequencies to a percentage. So, click 'Change' and then choose 'Analysis Parameter' and now check the boxes for 'Relative frequency' as well as 'Cumulative frequency'.

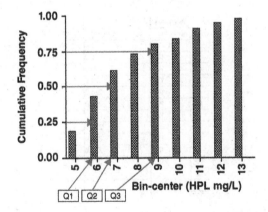

The Y axis is now in percentages, and the median and the interquartile range can be read from the X axis,

i.e.

- The first quartile (25%) is Q1.
- The third quartile (75%) or Q3.
- Thus, the interquartile range is Q3–Q1.
- The median is Q2.

Correlation Test

EXAMPLE 7.6 | To determine the correlation coefficient using Prism

---

The lactose content was measured in the milk produced by a herd of cows (Table 7.4).

TABLE 7.4 Lactose content and milk yield in cows

Cow	1	2	3	4	5	6	7	8	9	10
Lactose content (/g)	230	238	221	224	212	229	235	226	224	215
Milk Yield (/L)	18.6	19.6	17.3	18.2	16.4	19.1	20.0	17.7	18.6	17.3

a) State the regression equation

b) What is the lactose content in the milk of a cow which yields 18 litres?

Step 1: The data is first put into the spreadsheet, milk yield in the x column and lactose content in the Y column

	X Values	A	B
	milk yield/L	lactose content/g	Tit
	X	Y	Y
1	18.6	230.0	
2	19.6	238.0	
3	17.3	221.0	
4	18.2	224.0	
5	16.4	212.0	
6	19.1	229.0	
7	20.0	235.0	
8	17.7	226.0	
9	18.6	224.0	
10	17.3	215.0	
11			
12			

Step 2: Click 'Analyze' and then choose 'Statistical analysis' and 'Correlation' and click 'OK'

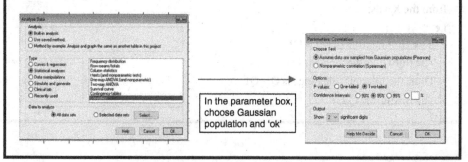

In the parameter box, choose Gaussian population and 'ok'

(continued)

EXAMPLE 7.6 *(continued)*

Step 3: Click on the 'Results' tab on the left

	Parameter	A lactose content/g Y
1	Number of XY Pairs	10
2	Pearson r	0.93◀
3	95% confidence interval	0.72 to 0.98
4	P value (two-tailed)	P<0.0001
5	P value summary	***
6	Is the correlation significant? (alpha=0.05	Yes
7	R squared	0.86
8		

The correlation coefficient r=0.93. This shows there is a strong relationship between milk yield and the lactose content

Regression Test

EXAMPLE 7.7 | Linear regression using Prism

Step 1: To obtain the regression equation, we need to do linear regression. Click on the 'Data' tab, then click 'Analyze', then choose 'Linear regression' from 'Curves & regression' and click 'OK'.

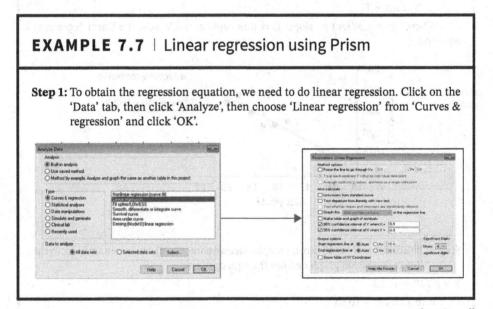

(continued)

EXAMPLE 7.7 (continued)

Step 2: Accept the choices in the parameter box and click 'OK'.

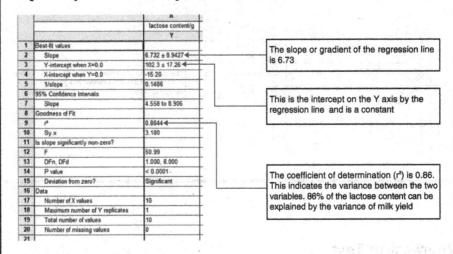

	A lactose content/g Y
1 Best-fit values	
2 Slope	6.732 ± 0.9427
3 Y-intercept when X=0.0	102.3 ± 17.26
4 X-intercept when Y=0.0	-15.20
5 1/slope	0.1486
6 95% Confidence Intervals	
7 Slope	4.558 to 8.906
8 Goodness of Fit	
9 r²	0.8644
10 Sy.x	3.180
11 Is slope significantly non-zero?	
12 F	50.99
13 DFn, DFd	1.000, 8.000
14 P value	< 0.0001
15 Deviation from zero?	Significant
16 Data	
17 Number of X values	10
18 Maximum number of Y replicates	1
19 Total number of values	10
20 Number of missing values	0
21	

The slope or gradient of the regression line is 6.73

This is the intercept on the Y axis by the regression line and is a constant

The coefficient of determination (r²) is 0.86. This indicates the variance between the two variables. 86% of the lactose content can be explained by the variance of milk yield

Step 3: Since the regression line is a straight line, and the equation for a straight line is 'Y = mx + C

Where, m = gradient or slope; C = intercept on the Y axis, the linear regression equation is:

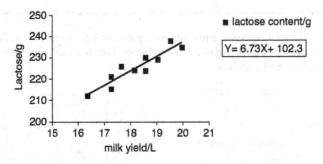

$Y = 6.73X + 102.3$

Step 4: If the milk yield is 18 litres, then the lactose content (Y) can be obtained from the linear regression graph or from the equation, i.e.

$Y = 6.73X + 102.3$

Or $Y = (6.73 \times 18) + 102.3$

Or $Y = 121.14 + 102.3$

Lactose content = 223.44/g

Student's t-test

EXAMPLE 7.8 | Paired t-test using Prism

The effect of a cholesterol-lowering drug taken daily for a month was tested on 12 volunteers (see Table 7.5). Plasma cholesterol was measured before and after treatment

TABLE 7.5   Levels of cholesterol before and after treatment

| Volunteer | Total Cholesterol (mmol/L) | |
	Pre-treatment	Post-treatment
1	6.0	5.7
2	6.5	6.2
3	5.3	5.0
4	5.4	5.3
5	6.2	6.0
6	5.5	5.1
7	5.8	5.0
8	5.4	5.2
9	6.0	5.4
10	6.1	5.7
11	6.1	5.8
12	5.9	5.5

a) Display the data for pre-treatment and post-treatment values as a bar graph
b) Select a suitable statistical test to assess whether the drug had a significant effect on plasma cholesterol levels.

Answer:

Step 1: Put the above data into the Prism spreadsheet in two Y columns

| | A | B |
| | pre-treatment | post-treatment |
	Y	Y
1	6.0	5.7
2	6.5	6.2
3	5.3	5.0
4	5.4	5.3
5	6.2	6.0
6	5.5	5.1
7	5.8	5.0
8	5.4	5.2
9	6.0	5.4
10	6.1	5.7

(continued)

EXAMPLE 7.8 (*continued*)

Step 2: Click 'Graphs' tab to see bar graphs of pre-treatment and post-treatment data.

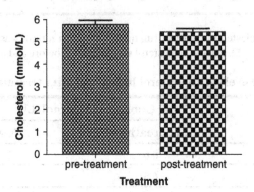

Step 3: As the same individuals were in the pre- and post-treatment groups a paired t-test was chosen.

Step 4: Slick the 'Data' tab, click 'Analyze', then 'Statistical analysis', and then 't-tests'.

Step 5: Select 'Data sets'.

Step 6: Select (in parameters choose 'Test (paired, two tail, CI)'.

Step 7: View tabular results.

	Parameter	Value
		Y
1	Table Analyzed	Data 2
2	Column A	pre-treatment
3	vs	vs
4	Column B	post-treatment
5		
6	Paired t test	
7	P value	0.0004
8	P value summary	***
9	Are means signif. different? (P < 0.05)	Yes
10	One- or two-tailed P value?	Two-tailed
11	t, df	t=5.5 df=9
12	Number of pairs	10
13		
14	How big is the difference?	
15	Mean of differences	0.36
16	95% confidence interval	0.21 to 0.51
17	R squared	0.77
18		
19	How effective was the pairing?	
20	Correlation coefficient (r)	0.88
21	P Value (one tailed)	0.0004
22	P value summary	***
23	Was the pairing significantly effective?	Yes
24		

The P value of 0.004 is much lower than 0.05, thus this is a significant result showing that cholesterol was lowered by the drug after 1 month

One-way ANOVA

This test is used to find differences in the mean for three or more sets of grouped data for a single factor, e.g. treatment, exercise, posture, reaction time. It is important to choose the correct ANOVA test (i.e. normal ANOVA). If the results show a significant difference then post-tests (Bonferroni, Tukey, Newman Keuls, Dunnett's) would be used to identify the pairings which show significance.

Step 1: In the empty data table, click 'New', then 'New Data Table, then the Create New Table box is shown

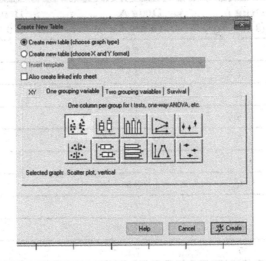

Step 2: Check 'Create new table', then click 'One grouping variable' and click 'Create'. Now type your data in the columns.

Step 3: After the data has been put in click 'Analyze', choose 'Statistical analysis', then 'One-way ANOVA'

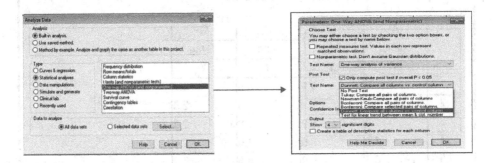

Step 4: Then fill in the parameters box for one-way ANOVA, including choosing a post ANOVA test to see which groups are significant if the ANOVA test shows significance.

EXAMPLE 7.9 | One-way ANOVA using Prism

The effect of different doses of a new steroid drug (drug A) on the level of pain perceived by patients with adhesive capsulitis (frozen shoulder) was tested on nine volunteers (Table 7.6).

TABLE 7.6	Pain scores in multiple sclerosis patients before and after drug A		
Control	Drug A (1 mg kg⁻¹)	Drug A (5 mg kg⁻¹)	Drug A (10 mg kg⁻¹)
10	9	5.5	4
8	7.5	4.5	2.5
9.5	6	6	2.5
7	5.5	4	2
8.5	6	6.5	3
7.5	7	5	4
9	6.5	5.5	5
8.5	7.5	7.0	3.5
8	8	6.7	3
9	7	7.1	3.7

a) Plot the data using an appropriate graphical format.

b) Select a suitable statistical test to assess whether drug A had an effect on frozen shoulder induced pain.

Answer

a) **Step 1:** Input the above data into 4 Y columns.

	A	B	C	D
	control	1mg	5mg	10mg
	Y	Y	Y	Y
1	10.0	9.0	5.5	4.0
2	8.0	7.5	4.5	2.5
3	9.5	6.0	6.0	2.5
4	7.0	5.5	4.0	2.0
5	8.5	6.0	6.5	3.0
6				

(continued)

EXAMPLE 7.9 (continued)

Step 2: Click on graph and using 'Change', improve the appearance of the graph.

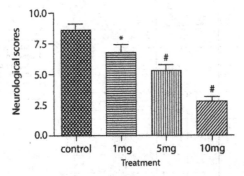

b) **Step 3:** A one factor analysis of variance (ANOVA) was chosen as the effect of dosage on pain was being investigated. In the data table, the Analyze tab is clicked, and 'One-way ANOVA' was chosen from 'Statistical analysis'.

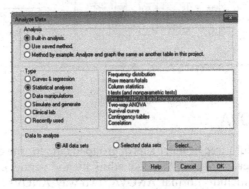

Step 4: From the parameters box, choose the 'One-way ANOVA', and the Dunnet's test as the post hoc test.

(continued)

EXAMPLE 7.9 (continued)

Step 5: Look at the generated results.

	Parameter	A Value	B Data Set-B	C Data Set-C	D Data Set-D
		Y	Y	Y	Y
1	Table Analyzed				
2	Data 5				
3	One-way analysis of variance				
4	P value	P<0.0001			
5	P value summary	***			
6	Are means signif. different? (P < 0.05)	Yes			
7	Number of groups	4			
8	F	23.39			
9	R squared	0.8143			
10					
11	Bartlett's test for equal variances				
12	Bartlett's statistic (corrected)	1.477			
13	P value	0.6876			
14	P value summary	ns			
15	Do the variances differ signif. (P < 0.05)	No			
16					
17	ANOVA Table	SS	df	MS	
18	Treatment (between columns)	90.34	3	30.11	
19	Residual (within columns)	20.60	16	1.288	
20	Total	110.9	19		
21					
22	Dunnett's Multiple Comparison Test	Mean Diff.	q	P value	95% CI of diff
23	control vs 1mg	1.800	2.508	P > 0.05	-0.05867 to 3.659
24	control vs 5mg	3.300	4.598	P < 0.01	1.441 to 5.159
25	control vs 10mg	5.800	8.082	P < 0.01	3.941 to 7.659

This shows a significant difference between control and the dosage of drug A. However, it does not tell us which dose is causing the significance. The post hoc test (Dunnett) lets you know which dose is effective

Drug A does show a significant reduction in pain for the 5mg and 10mg dose, but not for the 1mg dose

Two-way ANOVA

This test would be for three or more sets of grouped data for the effects of two factors or variables (e.g. treatment and exercise; ethnicity and gender). The types of ANOVA tests available include normal ANOVA, two-way ANOVA, repeated measures two-way ANOVA.

X labels	Before exercise	During exercise
Treatments		
None		
Drug A		
Drug B		

Again, you can directly set up the table and input data or clicking 'New', can set up new table. For two-way ANOVA, choose two grouping variables, as one factor variable is for the Y columns and the other factor is for the X columns.

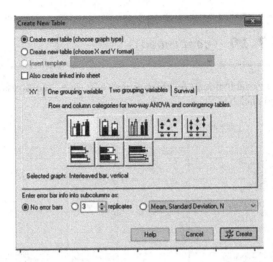

EXAMPLE 7.10 | Two-way ANOVA Using mean data

The effect of gender on salivary cortisol levels produced during a stress test (arithmetic test) was assessed in five males and five females between 9 am and 11 am. Cortisol was measured three times before the stress and at the end of the stress. The means and standard errors were calculated.

X Labels	A			B		
X Labels	Men			Women		
X	Mean	SEM	N	Mean	SEM	N
1 control	12.16	0.31	5	10.10	0.25	5
2 Stress	15.74	0.88	5	12.31	0.46	5
3						

a) Plot data graphically.
b) Does gender affect the stress response?

Step 1: First put data into data table in the data tab, click 'Analyze', then choose two-way ANOVA.

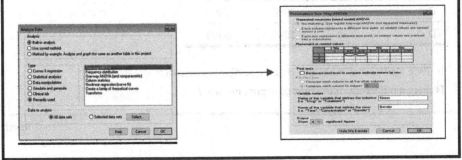

(continued)

EXAMPLE 7.10 *(continued)*

Step 2: Fill in the variable names for the columns and rows, here stress and gender was put in and click 'OK'.

Two-way ANOVA				
Source of Variation	% of total variation	P value		
Interaction	2.24	0.2186		
Stress	35.94	0.0001		
Gender	39.98	P<0.0001		
Source of Variation	P value summary	Significant?		
Interaction	ns	No		
Stress	***	Yes		
Gender	***	Yes		
Source of Variation	Df	Sum-of-squares	Mean square	F
Interaction	1	2.346	2.346	1.640
Stress	1	37.68	37.68	26.33
Gender	1	41.91	41.91	29.29
Residual	16	22.89	1.431	

Step 3: From the results we can see that the interaction between gender and stress is not significant, but both stress and gender show a significant effect on cortisol levels.

EXAMPLE 7.11 | Two-way ANOVA with raw data

The effect of three antibiotics (AB1, AB2, AB3) on inhibiting bacterial growth in four strains of the *Escherichia Coli* bacteria (A, B, C, D) was examined by measuring the minimum inhibitory concentrations (MIC) in μg/ml.

Strain	AB1	AB2	AB3
A	4000	8100	7985
B	4020	8005	7900
C	4056	7980	7880
D	2068	2080	3300

Is there a difference in the effect of the antibiotics on MIC?
Is there a difference in the type of strain and MIC?

(continued)

EXAMPLE 7.11 *(continued)*

Step 1: Put the above data into the data table of Prism.

	X Labels	A	B	C
	bac strains	AB1	AB2	AB3
	X	Y	Y	Y
1	A	4000	8100	7985
2	B	4020	8005	7900
3	C	4056	7980	7880
4	D	2068	2080	3300
5				

Step 2: Click 'Analyze' and choose 'Statistical Test' and highlight 'two-way ANOVA.

(continued)

EXAMPLE 7.11 *(continued)*

Step 3: Check the Bonferroni post-tests, check compare each column, put in the variable names for the rows and for the columns and click 'OK'. Note this is normal two-way ANOVA.

Parameters: Two-Way ANOVA

Repeated measures (mixed model) ANOVA

- ⦿ No matching. Use regular two-way ANOVA (not repeated measures).
- ◯ Each column represents a different time point, so related values are spread across a row.
- ◯ Each row represents a different time point, so related values are stacked into a subcolumn.

Placement of related values:

	X Title	Title		Title		Title	
	X	A:Y1	A:Y2	B:Y1	B:Y2	C:Y1	C:Y2
1							
2							
3							

Post tests

☑ Bonferroni post-tests to compare replicate means by row.

For each row:

- ⦿ Compare each column to all the other columns
- ◯ Compare each column to column A ⌄

Variable names

Name of the variable that defines the columns: Antibiotic
(i.e. "Drug" or "Treatment")

Name of the variable that defines the rows: bac strains
(i.e. "Time", "Concentration" or "Gender")

Output

Show 4 ⌄ significant figures

[Help Me Decide]   [Cancel]   [OK]

(continued)

EXAMPLE 7.11 (*continued*)

Step 4: The results below show there is a significant effect of bacterial strains and antibiotic on the MIC, but comparisons between antibiotics show no significance.

	Y	Y	Y	
Table Analyzed	Data 3			
Two-way ANOVA				
Source of Variation	% of total variation	P value		
Antibiotic	36.41	0.0071		
bac strains	54.90	0.0053		
Source of Variation	P value summary	Significant?		
Antibiotic	**	Yes		
bac strains	**	Yes		
Source of Variation	Df	Sum-of-squares	Mean square	F
Antibiotic	2	26020000	13010000	12.58
bac strains	3	39240000	13080000	12.64
Residual	6	6207000	1034000	
Number of missing values	-12			

Non-Parametric Tests

Wilcoxan test

EXAMPLE 7.12 | Wilcoxon non-parametric test

A group of nine women had their ventilation (L min^{-1}) measured during the follicular and luteal phase of the ovulatory cycle. Is there a difference in the ventilation between the two phases?

Subject	1	2	3	4	5	6	7	8	9
Follicular phase	8	10	9	14	12	9	11	10	13
Luteal phase	15	15	20	23	19	14	16	17	21

(*continued*)

EXAMPLE 7.12 (*continued*)

Step 1: Put the data into the Prism data sheet.

	A	B	
	Follicular	Luteal	
	Y	Y	
1	8	15	
2	10	15	
3	9	20	
4	14	23	
5	12	19	
6	9	14	
7	11	16	
8	10	17	
9	13	21	
10			

Step 2: Click 'Analyze', then choose 'Statistical analysis', and highlight 't-tests (and nonparametric)' and click 'OK'.

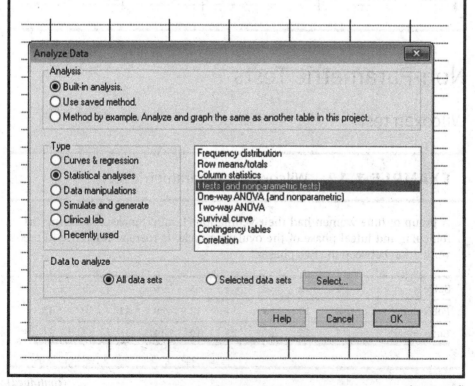

EXAMPLE 7.12 (*continued*)

Step 3: Check the boxes for Nonparametric test, choose Wilcoxon matched
pairs test, and click 'OK'.

Parameters: t Tests (and Nonparametric Tests)   ✕

Choose Test

You may either choose a test by checking the three option boxes, or
you may choose a test by name below.

☑ Paired test. Values in each row represent paired observations.

☑ Nonparametric test. Don't assume Gaussian distributions.

☐ Welch's correction. Don't assume equal variances.

Test Name: Wilcoxon matched pairs test   ⌄

Options

P values: ○ One-tailed   ◉ Two-tailed

Confidence Intervals: ○ 90% ◉ 95% ○ 99% ○ ☐ %

Output

Show 4 ⌄ significant digits

☐ Create a table of descriptive statistics for each column

Help Me Decide   Cancel   OK

(*continued*)

EXAMPLE 7.12 (*continued*)

Step 4: The results below show that there is a significant difference in the medians of the follicular and luteal phases.

	Parameter	A Value Y
1	Table Analyzed	Data 1
2	Column A	Follicular
3	vs	vs
4	Column B	Luteal
5		
6	Wilcoxon signed rank test	
7	P value	0.0039
8	Exact or approximate P value?	Gaussian Approximation
9	P value summary	**
10	Are medians signif. different? (P < 0.05)	Yes
11	One- or two-tailed P value?	Two-tailed
12	Sum of positive, negative ranks	0.0000 , -45.00
13	Sum of signed ranks (W)	-45.00
14		
15	How effective was the pairing?	
16	rs (Spearman, Approximation)	0.7131
17	P Value (one tailed)	0.0155
18	P value summary	*
19	Was the pairing significantly effective?	Yes

Mann–Whitney Test

EXAMPLE 7.13 | Mann–Whitney non-parametric test

A new skin patch containing capsaicin was compared to a skin patch containing an opioid to treat neck pain. Two groups (A and B) of subjects suffering from neck pain were matched for age and gender and asked to rate their pain on a scale from 1 (low) to

(continued)

EXAMPLE 7.13 (continued)

10 (high) before and after 24 hrs of using the patches. Is there a difference in the pain scores reported by the two groups?

Subject	1	2	3	4	5	6	7	8	9	10
Group A (capsaicin)	7	5	4	4	6	3	3	6	7	6
Group B (opioid)	6	5	6	7	5	4	5	7	8	

Step 1: Put the above data into the data table for Prism.

A	B	C
GP A capsaicin	GP B Opioid	Ti
Y	Y	Y
7	6	
5	5	
4	6	
4	7	
6	5	
3	4	
3	5	
6	7	
7	8	
6		

Step 2: Click the 'Analyze' tab and choose 'Statistical analysis' and 't-tests (and nonparametric)' and click 'OK'.

Analyze Data

Analysis
- ◉ Built-in analysis.
- ○ Use saved method.
- ○ Method by example. Analyze and graph the same as another table in this project.

Type
- ○ Curves & regression
- ◉ Statistical analyses
- ○ Data manipulations
- ○ Simulate and generate
- ○ Clinical lab
- ○ Recently used

Frequency distribution
Row means/totals
Column statistics
t tests (and nonparametric tests)
One-way ANOVA (and nonparametric)
Two-way ANOVA
Survival curve
Contingency tables
Correlation

Data to analyze
- ◉ All data sets
- ○ Selected data sets   Select...

Help   Cancel   OK

(continued)

EXAMPLE 7.13 (*continued*)

Step 3: Check 'Nonparametric test' and choose 'Mann–Whitney and click 'OK'.

Step 4: The result below shows there is no significance, i.e. the medians are the same.

Parameter	A Value
	Y
Table Analyzed	Data 2
Column A	GP A capsaicin
vs	vs
Column B	GP B Opioid
Mann Whitney test	
P value	0.3154
Exact or approximate P value?	Gaussian Approximation
P value summary	ns
Are medians signif. different? (P < 0.05)	No
One- or two-tailed P value?	Two-tailed
Sum of ranks in column A,B	87.50 , 102.5
Mann-Whitney U	32.50

Summary

- At the start of Prism, the welcome menu allows you to the choose the table format for putting your data in, including mean data and replicates.
- For each statistical task or problem Prism uses 5 tabs (Data, Info, Results, Graphs, Layout).
- The data tab shows the data in a column and row format whilst the graph tab shows an immediate graphical view of the data.
- Choosing the 'Analyze' button allows you to choose the parametric or non-parametric test.
- Re-analysis of data is extremely fast.
- It is very easy to switch between tabs particularly the Data, Results, and Graphs.
- The 'Change' button allows modifications in the table format and graphs.
- In graphs, double clicking on a part of the graph gives options for change.
- It is easy to import and export data with Excel, and to export graphs to Powerpoint.
- A wide variety of statistical tests (parametric and nonparametric) are available.

CHAPTER 8

Using SPSS
Descriptive and Inferential Statistics

Expected Learning Outcomes

- Explain the structure, layout and uses of SPSS.
- Enter data correctly into SPSS.
- Calculate descriptive statistics using SPSS.
- Analyse and Interpret inferential statistics using SPSS.

What is SPSS?

SPSS (Statistics Package for the Social Sciences) is a statistical software package widely used in universities. It is very large and allows a comprehensive exploration and analysis of data to advanced level. However, it can be cumbersome to use and graphical presentation of data may not be the best.

When you enter the package, you will see a spreadsheet, with columns and rows; the data view screen. A second sheet called the 'variable view' is used to define the variables. It is important that data is put in columns and variables are defined by names and categories of variables are defined by number labels, e.g. 1 for smokers and 2 for non-smokers.

Data Entry

1. Data is entered in the data editor screen ('SPSS Data Editor').
2. Data is entered in the worksheet called 'data view'. Data is entered in rows where each row represents a particular person and the variables are the column names. SPSS will only take numbers.

Essential Statistics for Bioscientists, First Edition. Mohammed Meah.
© 2022 John Wiley & Sons Ltd. Published 2022 by John Wiley & Sons Ltd.

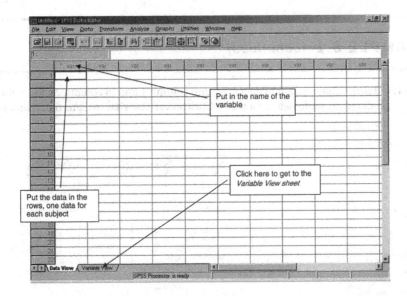

3. The worksheet called 'variable view' gives further information on the data; click on this to name the column variables and to specify which group is control and which is experimental. Groups have to be identified by using numbers (e.g. controls all have 1 and experimental group all have 2 in the rows).

Descriptive Statistics, Graphical Display, and Normality Testing Using SPSS

EXAMPLE 8.1 | Descriptive statistics, graphical display of data, histograms, test of normality

The haemoglobin concentration was measured from finger prick blood from 20 students (10 males and 10 females) and is shown in Table 8.1.

TABLE 8.1   **Hb in males and females**

Gender	Haemoglobin(g dl^{-1})
Female	15.00, 13.50, 13.00, 12.00, 11.50, 16.00, 15.40, 13.20, 14.20, 16.00
Male	14.00, 15.00, 13.60, 15.80, 16.70, 17.10, 14.70, 15.50, 17.30, 16.90

a. Calculate the descriptive statistics.
b. Show plots of box and whisker, histograms, stem and leaf.
c. Test the normality of the data for males and females (Kolmogorov–Smirnov test).

(continued)

EXAMPLE 8.1 *(continued)*

Step 1: Enter the above data into data view into column 1 and in column 2 specify the gender (e.g. 1 for female, 2 for male). Click on variable view to name the columns.

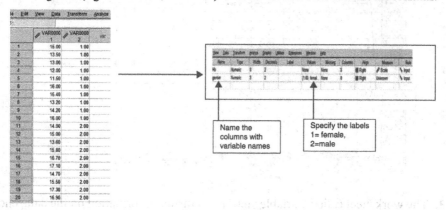

Name the columns with variable names

Specify the labels
1= female,
2=male

Step 2: Click on 'Analyse' menu, then 'Descriptive Statistics', then 'Explore'.

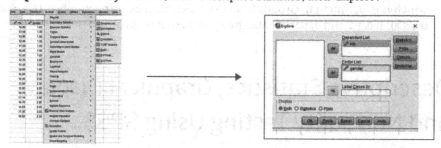

Step 3: Put 'Hb' into the 'Dependent List' box and gender into the 'Factor List'. Click 'Plots' and choose 'Histogram', 'Stem-and-leaf' and 'Normality plots with tests'.

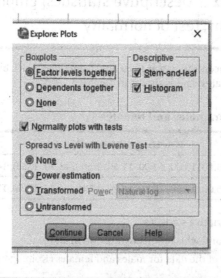

(continued)

EXAMPLE 8.1 *(continued)*

Step 4: Then click 'OK' and an output file window will open showing the descriptive statistics (mean, SD, SEM, 95% confidence interval for the mean) for both males and females plus tests of normality, histograms, stem and leaf plots, box and whisker plots as shown below.

Descriptive data for males and females:

Descriptives

gender			Statistic	Std. Error
Hb	female	Mean	13.9800	.50702
		95% Confidence Interval for Mean Lower Bound	12.8330	
		Upper Bound	15.1270	
		5% Trimmed Mean	14.0056	
		Median	13.8500	
		Variance	2.571	
		Std. Deviation	1.60333	
		Minimum	11.50	
		Maximum	16.00	
		Range	4.50	
		Interquartile Range	2.80	
		Skewness	-.139	.687
		Kurtosis	-1.268	1.334
	male	Mean	15.6600	.41879
		95% Confidence Interval for Mean Lower Bound	14.7127	
		Upper Bound	16.6073	
		5% Trimmed Mean	15.6833	
		Median	15.6500	
		Variance	1.754	
		Std. Deviation	1.32430	
		Minimum	13.60	
		Maximum	17.30	
		Range	3.70	
		Interquartile Range	2.43	
		Skewness	-.243	.687
		Kurtosis	-1.380	1.334

Box and Whisker Plots:

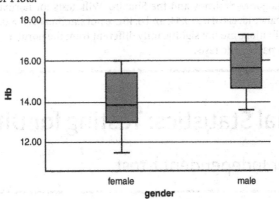

Stem and Leaf Plot:

```
Hb Stem-and-Leaf Plot for
gender= female
Frequency     Stem &  Leaf

     1.00       11 .  5
     1.00       12 .  0
     3.00       13 .  025
     1.00       14 .  2
     2.00       15 .  04
     2.00       16 .  00

Stem width:      1.00
Each leaf:       1 case(s)
```

(continued)

EXAMPLE 8.1 *(continued)*

Histogram Plots:

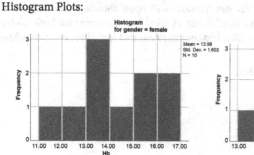

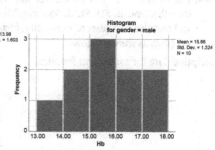

Tests for normality:

Tests of Normality

	gender	Kolmogorov-Smirnov[a]			Shapiro-Wilk		
		Statistic	df	Sig.	Statistic	df	Sig.
Hb	female	.138	10	.200[*]	.939	10	.543
	male	.184	10	.200[*]	.932	10	.465

*. This is a lower bound of the true significance.

a. Lilliefors Significance Correction

From the Kolmogorov–Smirnov and the Shapiro–Wilk tests for normality, we can see that the significance levels of 0.2, 0.54, and 0.46 are not significant ($P > 0.05$). This means that these distributions are not significantly different from the normal distributions and can be used for parametric tests.

Inferential Statistics: Testing for Differences

Unpaired or Independent t-test

EXAMPLE 8.2 | Unpaired t-test using spss

To test whether there is a difference between two sets of unpaired measurements, let us use the data from the previous example.

Gender	Haemoglobin(g dl⁻¹)
Female	15.00, 13.50, 13.00, 12.00, 11.50, 16.00, 15.40, 13.20, 14.20, 16.00
Male	14.00, 15.00, 13.60, 15.80, 16.70, 17.10, 14.70, 15.50, 17.30, 16.90

(continued)

EXAMPLE 8.2 *(continued)*

Step 1: Put all the data in the same column because each measurement is on a different person. In the second column to distinguish between the two groups use '1' for the first group and '2' for the second group.

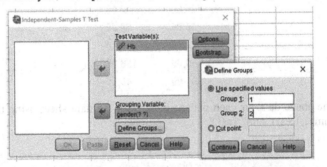

Step 2: Click 'Analyze', 'Compare Means', and 'Independent-Samples T-test'.

Step 3: Put variable name (Hb) in the 'Test variable(s)' box, and the subgroup (e.g. gender) in the 'Grouping Variable' box. In the 'Define Groups' box, put in the 1 and 2 used previously. Click on continue, then click 'OK'.

T-Test

Group Statistics

	gender	N	Mean	Std. Deviation	Std. Error Mean
Hb	female	10	13.9900	1.60333	.50702
	male	10	15.8600	1.32430	.41879

Independent Samples Test

		Levene's Test for Equality of Variances		t-test for Equality of Means					95% Confidence Interval of the Difference	
		F	Sig.	t	df	Sig. (2-tailed)	Mean Difference	Std. Error Difference	Lower	Upper
Hb	Equal variances assumed	.505	.454	-2.555	18	.020	-1.88000	.65761	-3.06158	-.29842
	Equal variances not assumed			-2.555	17.300	.020	-1.88000	.65761	-3.06512	-.29488

Step 4: From the results we can see that the Levene's test shows there is equal variance in the male and female groups since P > 0.05. Like the F-test, Levene's test is used to see whether there is equal variance or unequal variance in the groups The significance test for the means shows a significant difference in Hb between the males and females.

Paired t-test

EXAMPLE 8.3 | To test whether there is a difference be-
tween the means of two sets of paired measurements

A standard treatment (treat1) was compared to a new treatment (treat2) for varicose
ulcers in 12 matched pairs of patients, by measuring number of days from the start of
treatment to healing of the ulcer. This is shown below.

treat1	treat2
35.00	27.00
104.00	52.00
27.00	46.00
53.00	33.00
72.00	37.00
64.00	82.00
96.00	51.00
121.00	92.00
86.00	68.00
41.00	62.00
60.00	58.00
55.00	48.00

Step 1: The above data for each patient is put into the data sheet using the variable
names 'treat1' and 'treat2'.

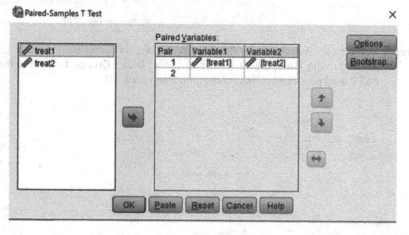

EXAMPLE 8.3 *(continued)*

Step 2: Click 'Analyze', 'Compare Means', and then 'Paired-Samples T-test' and the above box appears. Put variables to be compared (i.e. treat1 and treat2) – then click 'OK'.

Paired Samples Statistics

		Mean	N	Std. Deviation	Std. Error Mean
Pair 1	treat1	67.8333	12	28.92257	8.34923
	treat2	54.6667	12	19.23696	5.55323

Paired Samples Correlations

		N	Correlation	Sig.
Pair 1	treat1 & treat2	12	.538	.071

Paired Samples Test

		Paired Differences							
				Std. Error	95% Confidence Interval of the Difference				
		Mean	Std. Deviation	Mean	Lower	Upper	t	df	Sig. (2-tailed)
Pair 1	treat1 - treat2	13.16667	24.64598	7.11468	-2.49284	28.82597	1.851	11	.091

Step 3: The above results are produced. From this we can see that the significance (0.091) is greater than 0.05. Thus, there is no difference between the two types of treatment.

Correlation Test

EXAMPLE 8.4 | Association between data-correlation

In 15 individuals the lung function variable PEF (peak expiratory flow) in l min^{-1} was measured together with their height in cm (Table 8.2). Is there a relationship between these two variables.

TABLE 8.2 **PEF versus height**

PEF (l min^{-1})	Height (cm)
520	167
610	182
460	153
340	150
400	152
350	148
270	149
420	151

(continued)

EXAMPLE 8.4 *(continued)*

PEF (l min⁻¹)	Height (cm)
540	173
570	178
400	150
390	154
400	153
290	153
600	180

Step 1: The two columns of data were put into the data sheet.

Step 2: Click the 'Graphs' tab and then then choose 'Chart Builder'.

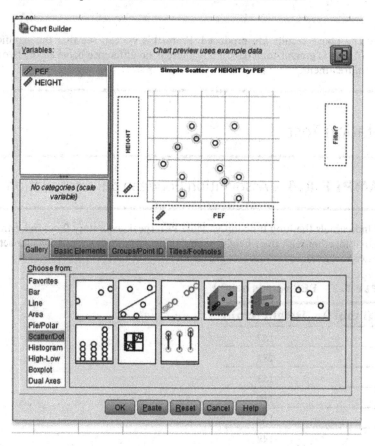

(continued)

EXAMPLE 8.4 *(continued)*

Step 3: Choose 'Scatter/Dot' from the Gallery menu. Then in the top window drag 'HEIGHT' and 'PEF' to the 'X' and 'Y' axis labels and click 'OK'.

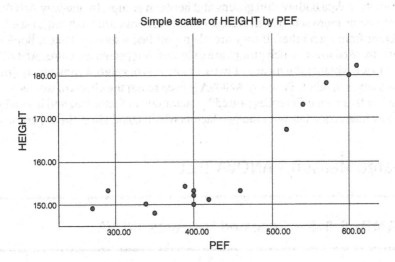

Simple scatter of HEIGHT by PEF

Step 4: A scatter plot of height against PEF is shown.

Step 5: Click 'Analyze', then choose 'Correlate', then 'Bivariate' correlations. A box will then appear called Bivariate Correlations. Move the PEF and Height labels to the small box called variables. Then tick 'Pearson', click the 'Two-tailed' button and tick 'Flag significant Correlations' then 'OK'

Correlations

		PEF	HEIGHT
PEF	Pearson Correlation	1	.912**
	Sig. (2-tailed)		.000
	N	15	15
HEIGHT	Pearson Correlation	.912**	1
	Sig. (2-tailed)	.000	
	N	15	15

**. Correlation is significant at the 0.01 level (2-tailed).

Step 6: From the analysis, we can see that there was a significant positive association between peak expiratory flow and height ($r = 0.912$, $P < 0.01$).

Testing for Differences between More than One Group

When there are multiple groups to compare differences, ANOVA is used to compare the variability of data both within groups and between groups. In one-way ANOVA the means of two or more sets of **unrelated measurements** are analysed to see if they are different from each other. If they are, then post hoc tests (e.g. Tukey, Bonferroni, Dunnett), are used to see which groups are different. A repeated measures ANOVA test is is used to see whether the means of two or more sets of **related measurements** are different from each other. Two-way ANOVA is used to test the effects of two factors. We test whether there are differences caused by factor one or factor two and also whether there is any interaction between the two factors which could affect the experiment.

Repeated Measures ANOVA Test

EXAMPLE 8.5 | Repeated Measures ANOVA

Eight subjects had their frequency of brain waves (alpha waves) measured in Hz in three conditions, control, music, and meditation. Which activities affected the production of alpha waves?

Step 1: Put the data into four different columns on the data sheet.

subject	control	music	meditation
1.00	15.00	12.00	9.00
2.00	12.00	10.00	11.00
3.00	20.00	15.00	12.00
4.00	35.00	25.00	19.00
5.00	30.00	26.00	17.00
6.00	31.00	20.00	20.00
7.00	25.00	19.00	15.00
8.00	11.00	18.00	13.00

Step 2: Click 'Analyze' tab and 'General Linear Model' then 'Repeated Measures'.

Analyze	Graphs	Utilities	Extensions	Window	Help

Reports ▶
Descriptive Statistics ▶
Bayesian Statistics ▶
Tables ▶
Compare Means ▶
General Linear Model ▶   Univariate...
Generalized Linear Models ▶   Multivariate...
Mixed Models ▶   Repeated Measures...
Correlate ▶   Variance Components...
Regression ▶

var   var   var

(continued)

EXAMPLE 8.5 *(continued)*

Step 3: In the box that appears, type in 'condition' to replace the 'factor1' for the 'Within-Subject Factor Name' and click in the 'Number of Levels box and put 3 (since this is the number of conditions). Now click 'Add' to confirm and then click 'Define'.

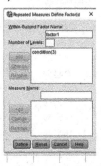

Step 4: Now move the three conditions to the 'Within-Subjects Variables', then click 'Options' and choose 'Descriptive statistics' which will generate means and standard deviations.

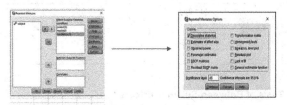

Step 5: Now click 'OK' to run the analysis. Shown below are the descriptive statistics, multivariate tests and Mauchly's tests of Sphericity.

The descriptive statistics show that the means decrease from control for music and meditation, suggesting there is an effect. Unless you are keen, you can ignore the multivariate tests and Mauchly's test.

Descriptive Statistics

	Mean	Std. Deviation	N
control	22.3750	9.22632	8
music	18.1250	5.69304	8
meditation	14.5000	3.92792	8

Multivariate Tests[a]

Effect		Value	F	Hypothesis df	Error df	Sig.
condition	Pillai's Trace	.709	7.300[b]	2.000	6.000	.025
	Wilks' Lambda	.291	7.300[b]	2.000	6.000	.025
	Hotelling's Trace	2.433	7.300[b]	2.000	6.000	.025
	Roy's Largest Root	2.433	7.300[b]	2.000	6.000	.025

a. Design: Intercept
   Within Subjects Design: condition

b. Exact statistic

Mauchly's Test of Sphericity[a]

Measure: MEASURE_1

					Epsilon[b]		
Within Subjects Effect	Mauchly's W	Approx. Chi-Square	df	Sig.	Greenhouse-Geisser	Huynh-Feldt	Lower-bound
condition	.621	2.855	2	.240	.725	.865	.500

Tests the null hypothesis that the error covariance matrix of the orthonormalized transformed dependent variables is proportional to an identity matrix.

a. Design: Intercept
   Within Subjects Design: condition

b. May be used to adjust the degrees of freedom for the averaged tests of significance. Corrected tests are displayed in the Tests of Within-Subjects Effects table.

(continued)

EXAMPLE 8.5 *(continued)*

Tests of Within-Subjects Effects

Measure: MEASURE_1

Source		Type III Sum of Squares	df	Mean Square	F	Sig.
condition	Sphericity Assumed	248.583	2	124.292	9.627	.002
	Greenhouse-Geisser	248.583	1.451	171.354	9.627	.007
	Huynh-Feldt	248.583	1.731	143.610	9.627	.004
	Lower-bound	248.583	1.000	248.583	9.627	.017
Error(condition)	Sphericity Assumed	180.750	14	12.911		
	Greenhouse-Geisser	180.750	10.155	17.799		
	Huynh-Feldt	180.750	12.117	14.917		
	Lower-bound	180.750	7.000	25.821		

Tests of Within-Subjects Contrasts

Measure: MEASURE_1

Source	condition	Type III Sum of Squares	df	Mean Square	F	Sig.
condition	Linear	248.063	1	248.063	13.626	.008
	Quadratic	.521	1	.521	.068	.801
Error(condition)	Linear	127.438	7	18.205		
	Quadratic	53.313	7	7.616		

Tests of Between-Subjects Effects

Measure: MEASURE_1
Transformed Variable: Average

Source	Type III Sum of Squares	df	Mean Square	F	Sig.
Intercept	8066.667	1	8066.667	75.289	.000
Error	750.000	7	107.143		

Step 6: We can now see the remainder of the analysis. The most important one here is the Tests of Within-Subjects Effects. This indicates in the last column that this is a significant result, that meditation and music do have an effect on brain wave frequency. The Within-Subject Contrasts and Between-Subject results can be ignored.

One-way ANOVA test

EXAMPLE 8.6 | One-Way ANOVA

The number of yeast cells surviving after incubation periods is shown below.

Tray	Number of yeast cells (cm⁻³)			
	control	24 hrs	30 hr	36 hrs
1	47	38	29	19
2	52	40	30	12
3	58	37	28	9
4	55	36	29	16
5	50	41	26	13

Are there any differences in survival of yeast cells between the incubation periods?

Step 1: Put above data into the data view spreadsheet. Put number of yeast cells in one column and the incubation periods as 1 for control, 2 for 24 hrs, 3 for 30 hrs and 4 for 36 hrs.

	yeastcel	ltime	var
1	47.00	1.00	
2	52.00	1.00	
3	58.00	1.00	
4	55.00	1.00	
5	50.00	1.00	
6	38.00	2.00	
7	40.00	2.00	
8	37.00	2.00	
9	36.00	2.00	
10	41.00	2.00	
11	29.00	3.00	
12	30.00	3.00	
13	28.00	3.00	
14	29.00	3.00	
15	26.00	3.00	
16	19.00	4.00	
17	12.00	4.00	
18	9.00	4.00	
19	16.00	4.00	
20	13.00	4.00	

(continued)

EXAMPLE 8.6 *(continued)*

Step 2: Go to variable view and under the 'values' tab for row 2, define the numbers 1, 2, 3, 4 as control, 24 hrs, 30 hrs, 36 hrs respectively. Then in data view click 'Analyze'.

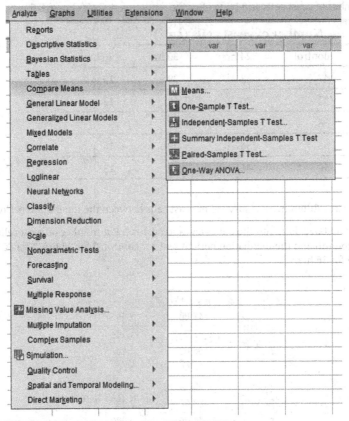

Step 3: Click 'Compare Means', then 'One-Way ANOVA'.

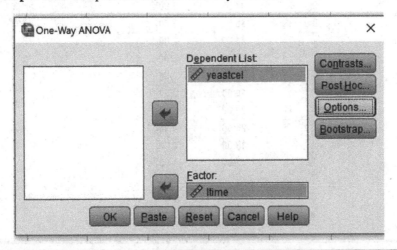

(continued)

EXAMPLE 8.6 *(continued)*

Step 4: Put the dependent variable (yeastcel) in the dependent list and independent variable (itime) in the factor box.

Step 5: Choose Descriptive statistics from options and from Post-Hoc choose tests to compare groups, e.g. Dunnetts.

Oneway

Descriptives

yeastcel

	N	Mean	Std. Deviation	Std. Error	95% Confidence Interval for Mean Lower Bound	Upper Bound	Minimum	Maximum
control	5	52.4000	4.27785	1.91311	47.0883	57.7117	47.00	58.00
24hr	5	38.4000	2.07364	.92736	35.8252	40.9748	36.00	41.00
30hr	5	28.4000	1.51658	.67823	26.5169	30.2831	26.00	30.00
36hr	5	13.8000	3.83406	1.71464	9.0394	18.5606	9.00	19.00
Total	20	33.2500	14.75011	3.29823	26.3467	40.1533	9.00	58.00

ANOVA

yeastcel

	Sum of Squares	df	Mean Square	F	Sig.
Between Groups	3975.350	3	1325.117	133.850	.000
Within Groups	158.400	16	9.900		
Total	4133.750	19			

Dunnett t (2-sided)[b]	control	36hr	38.60000*	1.98997	.000	33.4413	43.7587
	24hr	36hr	24.60000*	1.98997	.000	19.4413	29.7587
	30hr	36hr	14.60000*	1.98997	.000	9.4413	19.7587

*. The mean difference is significant at the 0.05 level.

b. Dunnett t-tests treat one group as a control, and compare all other groups against it.

Step 6: We can see there is a significant difference between groups. From the post hoc test by Dunnett, we can see that there are significant differences between the control and the other time durations for cell survival.

Two-way ANOVA test

EXAMPLE 8.7 | Two-way ANOVA

Nine males and nine females had their plasma glucose (mmol L⁻¹) measured before and after exercise (Table 8.3). What is the effect of exercise and gender on the plasma glucose?

TABLE 8.3 Glucose before and after exercise in males and females

Male control	Female control	Male exercise	Female exercise
5.7	4.8	4.9	4.1
5.2	5.2	5.3	4.9
5.1	5.5	4.8	4.8
5.8	5.2	5.0	5.1
5.3	4.9	4.8	4.5
5.0	5.3	4.5	4.8
5.5	5.0	5.0	5.2
6.1	5.5	5.2	4.3
5.5	4.8	4.9	4.5

Step 1: The above data is put into the data view. In this example we have two factors or independent variables, one is gender and the other is activity or exercise. To input this data first go to variable view and type in gender, glucose and exercise.

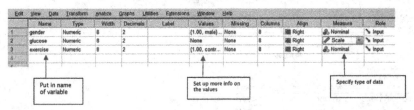

Step 2: Then click on cells under values and use 1 and 2 to label gender and activity.

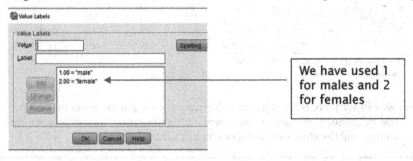

(continued)

EXAMPLE 8.7 *(continued)*

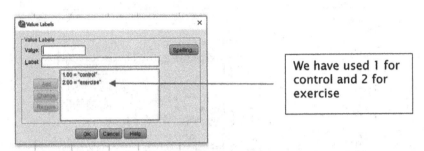

We have used 1 for control and 2 for exercise

Step 3: Now put nine 1 s and nine 2 s in the column labelled gender to represent male and female controls and similarly 1 s and 2 s in the exercise column to represent control and exercise. Then put in the values of glucose. Do check that the glucose values are assigned to the right group.

gender	glucose	exercise
2.00	5.20	2.00
2.00	4.90	2.00
2.00	5.30	2.00
2.00	5.00	2.00
2.00	5.50	2.00
2.00	4.80	2.00
1.00	4.90	1.00
1.00	5.30	1.00
1.00	4.80	1.00
1.00	5.00	1.00
1.00	4.80	1.00
1.00	4.50	1.00
1.00	5.00	1.00
1.00	5.20	1.00
1.00	4.90	1.00
2.00	4.10	2.00
2.00	4.90	2.00
2.00	4.80	2.00
2.00	5.10	2.00
2.00	4.50	2.00
2.00	4.80	2.00
2.00	5.20	2.00
2.00	4.30	2.00
2.00	4.50	2.00

Step 4: Now let us explore this data to see if they are normally distributed and if variances are equal to check that its OK to use parametric analysis. Click Analyse and choose 'Descriptive Statistics', then 'Explore'.

(continued)

EXAMPLE 8.7 *(continued)*

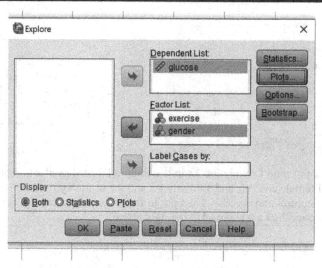

Step 5: Move the glucose to the 'Dependent List' and exercise and gender to the 'Factor List'. From Plots choose 'Histogram' then click 'OK'.

Descriptives

gender			Statistic	Std. Error
glucose	male	Mean	5.2000	.09463
		95% Confidence Interval for Mean — Lower Bound	5.0004	
		Upper Bound	5.3996	
		5% Trimmed Mean	5.1889	
		Median	5.1500	
		Variance	.161	
		Std. Deviation	.40147	
		Minimum	4.50	
		Maximum	6.10	
		Range	1.60	
		Interquartile Range	.60	
		Skewness	.589	.536
		Kurtosis	.185	1.038
	female	Mean	4.9111	.09143
		95% Confidence Interval for Mean — Lower Bound	4.7182	
		Upper Bound	5.1040	
		5% Trimmed Mean	4.9235	
		Median	4.9000	
		Variance	.150	
		Std. Deviation	.38789	
		Minimum	4.10	
		Maximum	5.50	
		Range	1.40	
		Interquartile Range	.48	
		Skewness	-.407	.536
		Kurtosis	-.222	1.038

(continued)

EXAMPLE 8.7 *(continued)*

Step 6: From the descriptive data, we can see that both the mean values for the male and female are similar. Variances are also similar. The medians are also very similar as can be seen in the box plots below.

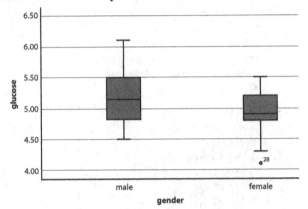

Step 7: When we consider the histograms, only two are shown below for male and female glucose levels. They could be normally distributed, however to confirm this we will do two common normality tests called the Kolmogorov–Smirnov and Shapiro–Wilk.

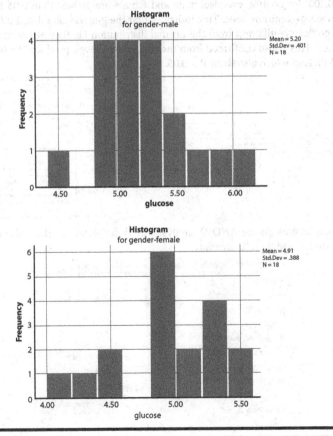

(continued)

EXAMPLE 8.7 *(continued)*

Step 8: To do the normality test, we click 'Analyze', choose 'Descriptive Statistics', then 'Explore' and a box will appear called Explore. Click 'Plots', then tick 'Normality plots with tests' and also 'Histogram', then 'Continue' and 'OK'.

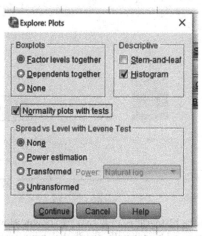

Step 9: From the results of the two normality tests, we can see that the significance levels (0.200) for control, exercise, male and female are greater than 0.05 for the Kolmogorov–Smirnov tests. This indicates that the glucose data distributions are not significantly different from the normal distribution i.e. they are normally distributed. This is also confirmed from the significance levels produced by the Shapiro–Wilk tests which also show P > 0.05.

Both the Kolmogorov-smirnov and Shapiro-Wilk normality tests show there is no significance P>0.05, so the glucose levels are not significantly different from the normal distribution and thus we can continue with parametric analysis.

Tests of Normality

		Kolmogorov-Smirnov[a]			Shapiro-Wilk		
	exercise	Statistic	df	Sig.	Statistic	df	Sig.
glucose	control	.151	17	.200	.951	17	.470
	exercise	.151	19	.200	.951	19	.412

*. This is a lower bound of the true significance.
a. Lilliefors Significance Correction

Note: If our data were not normally distributed, then we transform the data to see if normality can be achieved. You would need to click the 'Transform' tab then 'compute, put new variable name, then do a log transformation using LG10 (numexpr)

Step 10: Let us now do the ANOVA analysis. Click on 'Analyze', then 'General Linear Model' and then 'Univariate'.

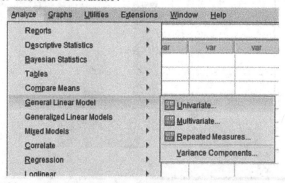

(continued)

EXAMPLE 8.7 *(continued)*

Step 11: In the box that appears, move glucose to Dependent Variable and gender and exercise to the Fixed factor boxes. Then click the 'Options' box on the right and tick 'Descriptive Statistics' and finally 'OK'.

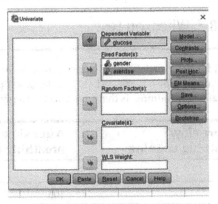

Step 12: The following analysis results are shown. As can be seen there is very little effect of exercise or gender on blood glucose glucose since the significances for both (0.158 and 0.442) are greater than 0.05.

Univariate Analysis of Variance

Between-Subjects Factors

		Value Label	N
gender	1.00	male	18
	2.00	female	18
exercise	1.00	control	18
	2.00	exercise	18

Descriptive Statistics

Dependent Variable: glucose

gender	exercise	Mean	Std. Deviation	N
male	control	5.2000	.40147	18
	Total	5.2000	.40147	18
female	exercise	4.9111	.38789	18
	Total	4.9111	.38789	18
Total	control	5.2000	.40147	18
	exercise	4.9111	.38789	18
	Total	5.0556	.41572	36

Tests of Between-Subjects Effects

Dependent Variable: glucose

Source	Type III Sum of Squares	df	Mean Square	F	Sig.
Corrected Model	.751[a]	1	.751	4.820	.035
Intercept	920.111	1	920.111	5905.076	.000
gender	.000	0			

(continued)

Non-parametric Tests

Wilcoxan Test

EXAMPLE 8.8 | Wilcoxon test

Ten subjects matched for their anxiety levels underwent slow breathing training three times a week for 30 minutes for 6 weeks. Their systolic blood pressure (mmHg) was measured before and after the training. Is there any effect of the slow breathing training?

Subject	Before slow breathing training	After slow breathing training
1	121	120
2	112	105
3	129	125
4	125	130
5	135	130
6	123	120
7	139	135
8	116	111
9	119	117
10	124	126

Step 1: Put the above data as two columns in data view.

Before	After	v
121.00	120.00	
112.00	105.00	
129.00	125.00	
125.00	130.00	
135.00	130.00	
123.00	120.00	
139.00	135.00	
116.00	111.00	
119.00	117.00	
124.00	126.00	

(continued)

EXAMPLE 8.8 *(continued)*

Step 2: Click 'Analyze' and then 'Nonparametric Tests' and then 'Related Samples'.

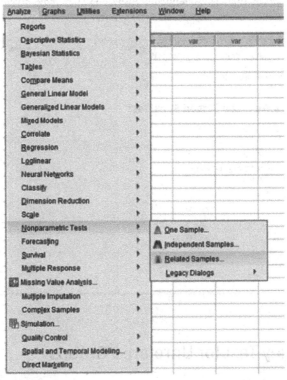

Step 3: In the non-parametric box, you have three tabs (Objective, Fields, Settings). If you leave it on the default, it will do more tests than you need, but that is not a problem. In the Field tab, you need to move your before and after variables to the test field. For the settings, you can customize and only tick Wilcoxons or leave it in default.

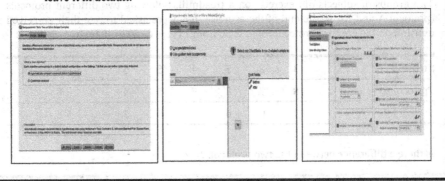

(continued)

EXAMPLE 8.8 *(continued)*

Step 4: From the results below, where differences in the median before and after have been compared, there is no significant difference (P = 0.082 > 0.05).

Hypothesis Test Summary

	Null Hypothesis	Test	Sig.	Decision
1	The median of differences between Before and After equals 0.	Related-Samples Wilcoxon Signed Rank Test	.082	Retain the null hypothesis.

Asymptotic significances are displayed. The significance level is .050.

Related-Samples Wilcoxon Signed Rank Test

Before, After

Related-Samples Wilcoxon Signed Rank Test Summary

Total N	10
Test Statistic	10.500
Standard Error	9.772
Standardized Test Statistic	-1.740
Asymptotic Sig (2-sided test)	.082

Mann–Whitney Test for Unrelated Groups

EXAMPLE 8.9 | Mann–Whitney test

Two groups of subjects did exercise on a treadmill, following two different protocols (protocol A and B). At the end of the exercise they were asked to rate their perceived exertion on the exercise protocols on a scale from 1 (very easy) to 10 (extremely hard).

Subject	1	2	3	4	5	6	7	8	9
Protocol A	8	7	8	7	5	9	8	8	7
Protocol B	7	6	6	7	8	5	7	6	

Is there a difference between the two protocols?

(continued)

EXAMPLE 8.9 *(continued)*

Step 1: Put all the perceived exertion data in one column. To distinguish between protocol A and protocol B, in the next column, put '1' for every data that is in protocol A and '2' for every data in protocol B.

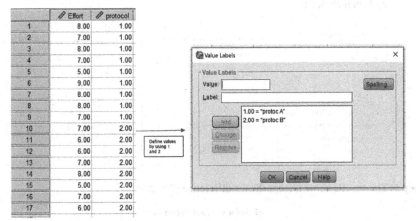

	Effort	protocol
1	8.00	1.00
2	7.00	1.00
3	8.00	1.00
4	7.00	1.00
5	5.00	1.00
6	9.00	1.00
7	8.00	1.00
8	8.00	1.00
9	7.00	1.00
10	7.00	2.00
11	6.00	2.00
12	6.00	2.00
13	7.00	2.00
14	8.00	2.00
15	5.00	2.00
16	7.00	2.00
17	6.00	2.00

Define values by using 1 and 2

Value Labels
Value:
Label:
1.00 = "protoc A"
2.00 = "protoc B"
Add   Change   Remove
OK   Cancel   Help

Step 2: Click on Variable view, then 'Value' for the second row, and define Field by stating what 1 and 2 represent. Click on the measure tab and define the data into nominal, ordinal and scale

Step 3: Click 'Analyze', then 'Nonparametric Tests', then 'Independent Samples'.

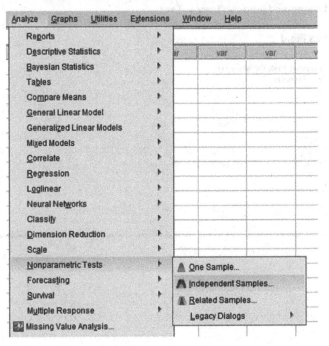

Analyze   Graphs   Utilities   Extensions   Window   Help
Reports
Descriptive Statistics
Bayesian Statistics
Tables
Compare Means
General Linear Model
Generalized Linear Models
Mixed Models
Correlate
Regression
Loglinear
Neural Networks
Classify
Dimension Reduction
Scale
Nonparametric Tests   One Sample...
Forecasting   Independent Samples...
Survival   Related Samples...
Multiple Response   Legacy Dialogs
Missing Value Analysis...

(continued)

EXAMPLE 8.9 *(continued)*

Step 4: For the Objective tab, leave on automatic; for the Field tab, make sure the variable is in the 'Test Fields' and the 'Field' is in the group box; For the settings, you can choose customise and then tick Mann–Whitney or leave on automatic, and then click Run.

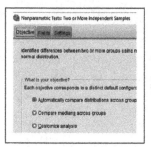 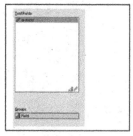 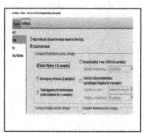

Step 5: The results show no significant difference (P > 0.05).

Hypothesis Test Summary

	Null Hypothesis	Test	Sig.	Decision
1	The distribution of protocol is the same across categories of Field.	Independent-Samples Mann-Whitney U Test	.074[a]	Retain the null hypothesis.

Asymptotic significances are displayed. The significance level is .050.

a. Exact significance is displayed for this test.

Independent-Samples Mann-Whitney U Test

protocol across Field

Independent-Samples Mann-Whitney U Test Summary

Total N	17
Mann-Whitney U	17.000
Wilcoxon W	53.000
Test Statistic	17.000
Standard Error	10.003
Standardized Test Statistic	-1.899
Asymptotic Sig.(2-sided test)	.058
Exact Sig. (2-sided test)	.074

Kruskall–Wallis test

EXAMPLE 8.10 | Kruskall–Wallis Test (non-parametric one-way ANOVA)

Students in one module were split into three groups based on an anxiety scale and were assessed in an oral presentation. The scores they obtained out of 100 are shown below:

No anxiety: 55, 66, 70, 57, 80

Moderate anxiety: 45, 40, 53, 57, 55

High anxiety: 40, 33, 30, 47, 38, 42

Is there any difference between the groups in the scores obtained in their oral presentations?

Step 1: Go to data view, and put the data of the marks in one column, and in the next column use the numbers 1, 2, and 3 to define the groups (no anxiety, moderate anxiety, and high anxiety).

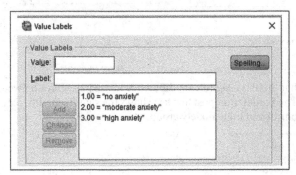

	Marks	groups
1	55.00	1.00
2	66.00	1.00
3	70.00	1.00
4	57.00	1.00
5	80.00	1.00
6	45.00	2.00
7	40.00	2.00
8	53.00	2.00
9	57.00	2.00
10	55.00	2.00
11	40.00	3.00
12	33.00	3.00
13	30.00	3.00
14	47.00	3.00
15	38.00	3.00

Step 2: Go to Variable view and define the values of the groups.

Step 3: Click 'Analyze', then 'Nonparametric Tests' and then 'Independent Samples'.

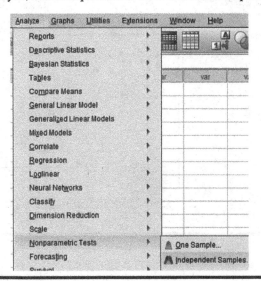

(continued)

EXAMPLE 8.10 *(continued)*

Step 4: Put 'Marks' in the Test Field and 'groups' into Groups. From tests choose Kruskal–Wallis and then run.

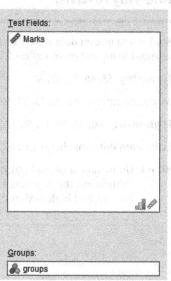

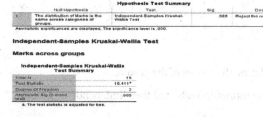

Step 5: The results show that there is a significant difference in median scores between
groups (P < 0.05). The Bonferrroni post hoc test shows the significant difference
was between the control and high anxiety group.

Hypothesis Test Summary

	Null Hypothesis	Test	Sig.	Decision
1	The distribution of Marks is the same across categories of groups.	Independent-Samples Kruskal-Wallis Test	.005	Reject the null hypothesis.

Asymptotic significances are displayed. The significance level is .050.

Independent-Samples Kruskal-Wallis Test

Marks across groups

Independent-Samples Kruskal-Wallis Test Summary

Total N	15
Test Statistic	10.411ᵃ
Degree Of Freedom	2
Asymptotic Sig. (2-sided test)	.005

a. The test statistic is adjusted for ties.

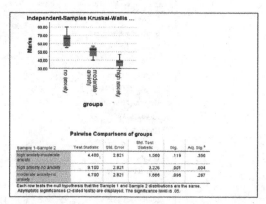

Pairwise Comparisons of groups

Sample 1-Sample 2	Test Statistic	Std. Error	Std. Test Statistic	Sig.	Adj. Sig.ᵃ
high anxiety-moderate anxiety	4.400	2.821	1.560	.119	.356
high anxiety-no anxiety	9.100	2.821	3.226	.001	.004
moderate anxiety-no anxiety	4.700	2.821	1.666	.096	.287

Each row tests the null hypothesis that the Sample 1 and Sample 2 distributions are the same.
Asymptotic significances (2-sided tests) are displayed. The significance level is .05.

Friedman Test

EXAMPLE 8.11 | Friedman Test (equivalent of the repeated measues ANOVA)

Twelve students who completed three level 4 modules in the first semester of their bioscience degree, were asked to complete an end of module satisfaction survey using a Likert Scale (1 = strongly disagree to 5 = strongly agree). Is there any difference in satisfaction between the modules?

Subject	Chemistry	Physiology	Biochemistry
1	3	4	4
2	5	4	3
3	2	3	4
4	1	2	2
5	4	2	4
6	4	5	4
7	3	4	3
8	5	3	3
9	4	4	4
10	3	3	3
11	3	4	4
12	4	4	4

Step 1: In the data view put in the above data in columns.

	Chemistry	Physiology	Biochemistry
1	3.00	4.00	4.00
2	5.00	4.00	3.00
3	2.00	3.00	4.00
4	1.00	2.00	2.00
5	4.00	2.00	4.00
6	4.00	5.00	4.00
7	3.00	4.00	3.00
8	5.00	3.00	3.00
9	4.00	4.00	4.00
10	3.00	3.00	3.00
11	3.00	4.00	4.00
12	4.00	4.00	4.00

(continued)

EXAMPLE 8.11 *(continued)*

Step 2: Click 'Analyze', then 'Nonparametric Tests', 'Legacy Dialogues' and 'K Related Samples'.

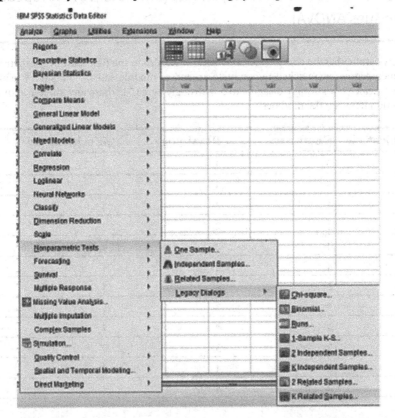

Step 3: Move the variables to the Test Variables box, and click 'Friedman' for the test type. Click 'Statistics' and tick the descriptive and quartile options, click 'Continue' and then 'OK'.

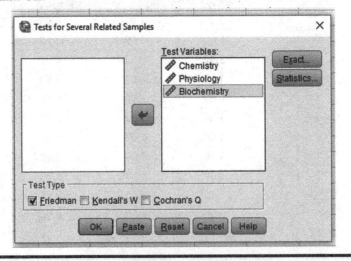

(continued)

EXAMPLE 8.9 *(continued)*

Step 4: The results below show that there is no significant difference between the mean ranks (P = 0.485) and thus no post hoc tests are required.

Descriptive Statistics

	N	Mean	Std. Deviation	Minimum	Maximum	25th	Percentiles 50th (Median)	75th
Chemistry	12	3.4167	1.16450	1.00	5.00	3.0000	3.5000	4.0000
Physiology	12	3.5000	.90453	2.00	5.00	3.0000	4.0000	4.0000
Biochemistry	12	3.5000	.67420	2.00	4.00	3.0000	4.0000	4.0000

Friedman Test

Ranks

	Mean Rank
Chemistry	1.79
Physiology	2.17
Biochemistry	2.04

Test Statistics[a]

N	12
Chi-Square	1.448
df	2
Asymp. Sig.	.485

a. Friedman Test

Summary

- SPSS uses the data tab to put in data and the variable tab to define the variables.
- Variable names are always put at the top of column.
- To define variables (particularly independent variables), numbers are used instead of names, e.g. males = 1 and females = 2. Sometimes you have to specify the type of data, e.g. nominal, ordinal, scalar.
- The 'Analyze' button is used for all analysis.
- The 'Explore' option allows calculation of descriptive statistics and various graphs.
- Frequency histograms can be shown from the sample data and be normalized or tested for normality.
- The general linear model is used to calculate differences between groups and association between groups.

CHAPTER 9

Misuse and Misinterpretations of Statistics

"There are three types of lies – lies, damn lies and statistics."

Benjamin Disraeli (1804–1881), 19th Century British Prime Minister (also attributed to Mark Twain.)

Expected Learning Outcomes

- Recognise common misinterpretations of statistical analysis.
- Explain factors that could affect data collection and interpretation.
- Minimize potential errors affecting experiments.

The final chapter of this book is going to briefly consider a very controversial and yet extremely important area which is the misuse of statistics in research whether intentional or not and how this can have major impacts on peoples' lives. In statistics we are collecting, displaying, and interpreting data. This data can be useful for a variety of purposes (e.g. census data for future planning of resources; survey data for marketing; research data for advancing knowledge and therapy). However, data can also be misused and manipulated (e.g. selective data in advertising and marketing of goods and services; access, storage and use of personal data in social media; non-disclosure of data due to commercial or other interests). I will now consider this misuse in relation to research in the biosciences.

What is Misuse of Statistics?

So what do I mean by misinterpretation and misuse of statistics. I am referring to the following:

- Errors in analysing data.
- Using statistical terms/language which reduces the ability for others to understand.

Essential Statistics for Bioscientists, First Edition. Mohammed Meah.
© 2022 John Wiley & Sons Ltd. Published 2022 by John Wiley & Sons Ltd.

- Publication of research which may be in error.
- Falsifying of research data.
- Misleading the public about the findings of the research.
- Being selective about research findings for gain.
- Presenting data in such a way as to mislead.
- Not declaring self-interests which will have an impact on research outcomes.

Computer software programs can be amazing tools to analyse data with their speed and their number crunching power. However, the old adage still applies about treating results with caution. The guidance provided by statistical software in choosing an appropriate test and interpreting the results varies widely depending on the name of the software. An additional problem is that the versions of software change frequently, and so there are compatibility issues in file recognition or instructions. Clearly more guidance is required in interpreting the statistical output, not necessarily from the software programs themselves.

Statistics is not an easy subject to understand or to apply easily in research. The majority of researchers do not have specialist knowledge of statistics and, therefore, there is the likelihood of statistical errors in manuscripts which may or may not be spotted. So it is not surprising to me that many journals receiving manuscripts lack the scrutiny of a statistician as is warranted. Adding to this is the pressure of the volume of manuscripts and the pressure to publish.

Implications From Clinical Research

Below are two examples which illustrate the impact of research particularly in a clinical area having major repercussions.

Dr Andrew Wakefield and colleagues published a paper in the Lancet in 1998, where he proposed a link between MMR (Measles, Mumps, and Rubella vaccine) vaccination and autism. This study was done in the Department of Paediatric Gastroenterology at the Royal Free Hospital. The impact of the publication led to patients questioning the safety of the vaccine, which led to a drop in the vaccination rate in the UK. He was investigated by the GMC (General Medical Council) which identified a number of faults in his study.

The GMC reported that he had a number of errors in his research design as well as ethical issues. He used children who were showing signs of autism and only 12 children were in the study. He carried out extra procedures such as lumber punctures and colonoscopies which weren't required; he did not declare conflict of interest although he had financial interests in the outcome of the study. No other studies showed a link between autism and the MMR vaccine. He was eventually struck off the medical register.

Mrs Sally Field was convicted of murdering her two children who died from SIDS (Sudden Infant Death Syndrome). One was 11 weeks old and the other was 8 weeks old. Professor Roy Meadows who was called as an expert witness said the risk of two babies dying was 1 in 73 million. Mrs Field served three years in prison, was released in 2003 and died in 2007. The Royal Statistical Society said the risk was 1 in 100 or 1 in 8500, i.e. much lower, so Professor Meadows calculations were in error.

The above two cases are important, because they illustrate in Dr Wakefield's case, the lack of scrutiny, poor design of the study and the attempts to mislead, whilst in Mrs Field's case we have an innocent woman who was at the mercy of a statistical misinterpretation, presented in court by a highly qualified professor.

What can we do to reduce the problems outlined above? Clearly, there is no instant panacea and we must be vigilant. We need institutions to strengthen and modify existing quality procedures where identified. We need more statisticians and training in universities and elsewhere to give more guidance and scrutiny. Above all, we need individuals to be their own regulator and follow ethical principles. With this regard, I would like to focus on experiments and how we can reduce some of the problems in carrying out research.

> **"Facts are stubborn things, but statistics are pliable."**
> *Samuel Langhorne Clemens, better known by his pen name Mark Twain (1835–1910), American author and humourist*

Factors Affecting the Results of Experiments

Samples

Some studies have a very small sample size and yet big conclusions are made as mentioned above. This is of crucial importance since any conclusions from the small sample may not be valid if applied to the population or for clinical diagnostic or therapy purposes. There is less confidence in the data and it may be difficult to publish the data.

As we have mentioned previously, in general, a large sample size is very important to the power of a study and for reducing the size of the confidence interval to make a better prediction of the population mean and thereby avoid a Type 2 error (assuming a non-significant result). However, there are some cases where small size samples may be valid (Bland 2009) particularly in the use of the t-test. If the sample size decreases to below six it is not possible to show significance ($P < 0.05$) between two groups using non-parametric methods such as Wilcoxon's, Mann–Witney, sign test, and this also applies to Spearman's and Kendall's rank correlation. The t-test may still be valid if the correlation between the two measurements is high (de Winter 2013).

Variation and Bias

In an experiment, subjects can react differently to an intervention, this is called inter-subject (between subjects) and intra-subject (within subject) variation. This is difficult to reduce, however, choosing a suitable experimental design, repetition and using replicates can help. Variability is greater when measurements are made on different subjects compared to within subject. This variation between independent groups can be reduced by matching characteristics such as age, gender, and severity of disease. Making too many measurements on the same subject can also be a problem (e.g. measuring blood pressure from both the left and right arms) if the results are pooled. The problems are that there is more likelihood of significance (Type 1 error) with increase in sample size from the pooling and that the samples are not independent (since the data is coming from the same subject).

Random variation is differences in results which cannot be explained. Factors that can cause random variation include, age, gender, ethnicity, medical history, state of health and unknown reasons. In an experimental design it is possible that another variable, called a confounding variable, has not been taken into account and could be affecting the experiment. Then it is difficult to have confidence that it is the independent variable which is the main intervention.

Bias is any influence which distorts the outcome, so conclusions are in error.

Randomized allocation of treatments or subjects may reduce bias. This can be simple randomization (e.g. each person is given an odd or an even number, all the patients allocated odd numbers would do experiment one and those allocated even numbers would do experiment two) or block randomization (e.g. 10 subjects grouped into two blocks for experiment A and B). We have already mentioned the importance of blinding and using placebo in designs to reduce bias in clinical trials.

Another aspect is bias in the publication of research. Studies with positive results (statistically significant result) tend to be published more than those with negative results; studies with positive conclusions are cited more frequently; a pharmaceutical company may withhold results which don't favour them; studies not written in English may not be included. So in effect the end result is we have missing publications. This is particularly important in clinical trials involving treatments, since published papers will be overrepresented in large trials and underrepresented in small trials in meta-analysis. One method of checking for publication bias is to examine funnel plots (see Chapter 2).

Reliability and Validity

Reliability refers to the consistency (precision) of a test or measurement and validity refers to the accuracy of the test or measurement. Both of these are essential in judging the quality of the research. In measurements we would like to be confident that we can rely on the test. So if we repeated the test the result will be within a certain percentage. For example the coefficient of variation for the repeat-test to be within ± 5%. Similarly, with our validity, frequent calibration would be carried out before, during, or after measurement to check accuracy or using positive and negative controls. A valid test should be reliable as well, ideally.

Presentation/reporting of Research Data

The publication of information from research can be presented in ways to favour the agenda of the person, body, or company. This includes being

- Selective with the data that is presented.
- Showing data in misleading graphs which include distortion of scales on y axis and not showing the baseline and.
- Showing data which describes a trend when collected on different groups, but when the groups are combined, the trend is reversed.

Statistical Analysis

Not choosing an appropriate statistical test to analyse data can lead to errors. For example, errors of significance such as Type 1 error (showing significance when there isn't any) or Type 2 error (showing no significance when there is). It is important that the criteria for tests (such as normality, variance of groups) are adhered to, however, it is recognised that there are robust-tests (such as the t-test) which allows some flexibility.

Correlation is often misused, particularly in clinical situations, as correlation between two variables does not imply causation. A *Lancet* study which showed a strong correlation between a low carbohydrate diet and lifespan said that it could lead to a shorter lifespan but did not take into account the quality of the food being consumed by the volunteers.

Suggestions for Reducing Errors in Experiments and in Reporting Experiments

It is important to scrutinize the research proposal, particularly in the experimental design to increase accuracy (expected value) and precision (repeatability) of the study.

This could include:

- Making sure equipment is regularly calibrated.
- Ensuring the calibration curve is linear (with correlation coefficient > 0.96).
- Using controls and standards (check that the coefficient of variation is under 5%).
- Using replicates in procedures (ideally three), e.g. three attempts.
- Checking the percentage error is low ((value measured - expected or quoted value)/expected value)x100).
- Having a large sample size, matching the groups or samples, or randomization.
- Having a consistent protocol to account for temperature variation, time of day, and calibration, to name a few.
- Being honest and ethical and declaring any self-interests.

> "If we are uncritical we shall always find what we want: we shall look for, and find, confirmations, and we shall look away from, and not see, whatever might be dangerous to our pet theories. In this way it is only too easy to obtain what appears to be overwhelming evidence in favour of a theory which, if approached critically, would have been refuted"
> – *Karl Popper (1902–1994) - Austrian-British philosopher*

Summary

- Misinterpretation and misuse of statistics refers to falsifying data, errors in analysing and presenting data.
- In all research studies it is important to rule out bias and to improve reliability (accuracy) and validity (precision).

- More planning needs to be done in designing studies, for example the sample size required, the protocol and experimental design and the methods of analysis. Is there a justification for the research? Are the outcomes achievable by the intended methods? Have ethical concerns been met?
- Reporting of studies should be in the scientific interest to advance knowledge and applications and not for self-interest or commercial purposes. Statistical findings should be reported and presented to avoid misinterpretation.

Appendix 1

Historical Landmarks in Statistics

Babylon, China, and India: recorded population data. Rulers needed information on resources (lands, agriculture, commerce, people) so that it could be used for taxation and for military campaigns. This was the earliest use of statistical data.

Roman Empire: made extensive records of the resources of the empire. They counted adult males, property, and population data.

Athenians: carried out censuses during both war and famine to assess resources.

Middle ages: saw extensive registration of land ownership and manpower. William the Conqueror (1028–1087), King of England, ordered the compilation of the *The Doomsday Book* of population and resources in England and Wales. Another example was the detailed censuses which were carried out in Paris in the 13th and 14th Centuries. These documented extensive detail of the Paris population, particularly, the taxes paid by individuals.

16th century: Girolamo Cardano (1501–1576), an Italian Mathematician: wrote *Liber de Ludo Aleae*, the first study of the principles of probability.

17th century: John Graunt (1620–1674), English statistician, William Petty (1623–1687), English economist, Blaise Pascal (1623–1662), French statistician and Daniel Bernoulli (1700–1782), Swiss mathematician: investigated statistics of populations (demography) and developed probability theory through games of chance and gambling.

Chevalier de Mere (1607–1684), gambler and French writer, made important contributions to probability theory from gambling with dice.

Blaise Pascal (1623–1662), also, laid foundations to mathematical theory of probability, binomial distribution and Pascal's triangle.

Abraham De Moivre (1667–1754), a French mathematician: worked on the normal distribution and probability theory, and equations of the normal curve. He worked on binomial predictions (e.g., heads or tails in tossing a coin) which led to the development of the normal distribution. Based on gambling in card games, dice, and roulette he calculated probabilities, including permutations and combinations. He also developed mortality tables and life insurance.

18th century: Pierre-Simon Marquis de Laplace (1749–1827), French mathematician: his work led to the early development of Bayesian Statistics and to the analytical theory of probability (central limit theorem).

James Lind (1716–1794), a doctor: did the first ever clinical trial in 1747 to find a treatment for scurvy using citrus fruits.

Gottfriend Achenwall (1719–1772), a German philosopher: first introduced the word 'Statistics'.

Essential Statistics for Bioscientists, First Edition. Mohammed Meah.
© 2022 John Wiley & Sons Ltd. Published 2022 by John Wiley & Sons Ltd.

19th century: Lambert Quatelet (1796–1874), a Belgian statistician, and Francis Galton (1822–1911), an English anthropologist: applied statistical analysis to human biology and genetics variation, in relation to anthropometry, intelligence (eugenics) and the concept of the 'average man'. Francis, also developed the concepts of standard deviation, correlation, and regression.

Carl Friedrich Gauss, a mathematician: developed the method of least squares in 1809. In 1821, he was the first to recognize the importance of the degree of freedom, which was defined and popularized by the statisticians William Gosset (also known as 'Student') and Ronald Fischer.

Florence Nightingale (1820–1910), British Nurse: Used statistics in tackling health problems and contributed to public health practice.

Charles Peirce (1839–1914), American philosopher: made major contributions to logic and introduced blinded, controlled randomized experiments.

20th century: Karl Pearson (1857–1936), English mathematician: developed the idea of correlation among variables. He founded, in 1911, a statistics department in University College. Pearson was the founder of mathematical statistics, natural selection using correlation, and developed Chi Squared analysis.

William Gossett (1876–1937): studied brewing, problems of small samples and developed the Student's t-test.

Carlo Bonferroni (1890–1960), Italian mathematician: Invented the 'Bonferroni Correction' for multiple comparisons and worked on probability.

Frank Wilcoxon (1892–1965), American chemist: developed the non-parametric Wilcoxon rank and sign tests.

Ronald Fisher (1890–1962), British biologist: laid the foundations for modern statistical science, developed ANOVA and highlighted the importance of randomization in experimental design, by considering growth of crops in fields and altering the conditions.

Charles Spearman (1863–1945), English psychologist: developed the non-parametric equivalent of correlation coefficient called the rank correlation.

Maurice Kendall (1907–1983), British statistician: also developed another non-parametric equivalent of the correlation coefficient.

JohnTukey (1915–2000), American statistician: developed a post hoc multiple comparisons procedure. He also developed the concept of exploratory data analysis, which included visualization of data graphically.

Charles Dunnett (1921–2007), Canadian Statistician: developed another multiple comparison procedure.

Matthijs Keuls, a Dutch horticulturist: also developed one, called the Newman-Keuls test in 1952.

Appendix 2

Common Statistical Terms

Analysis of Variance (ANOVA): statistical test to compare differences in more than two groups of data.

Biostatistics or Biometry: statistics applied to biological and medical sciences.

Cluster sampling: divide population into clusters.

Chi-squared: to test for differences between real and expected frequencies.

Confidence interval (95%) for the mean (CI): gives the values between which there is 95% confidence of finding the mean.

Class: data values split into groups.

Coefficient of determination (r^2): is the square of the correlation coefficient and gives an indication of the contribution one variable towards the other where there is a relationship between two variables.

Confounding factors: experimenter not able to distinguish between effects of different factors.

Continuous data: such as height and weight can be broken down to very small steps, such as decimals and thus provide more information.

Continuous variables: measure objects or attributes,area, volume, length, weight, temperature.

Correlation Coefficient (r): is a measure of the degree of relationship between two variables (value between −1 and +1).

Cross-sectional study: data collected at one point in time.

Critical values: predicted values of distributions which must be exceeded to show significance.

Data: units of information, such as numbers, words, observations, and measurements, can be quantitative or qualitative.

Degrees of freedom: the number of variables (independent variables) that you can manipulate, normally, it is sample size minus 1.

Dependent variable: the variable which is affected by the condition, intervention or manipulation of another variable (the independent variable).

Descriptive statistics: summarizing central and spread of values in sample data.

Discontinuous data: such as whole numbers, ranks, scales provide less information.

Discrete variable: fixed numbers (no decimals or fractions).

Error bars: bars drawn with mean data to show variation of standard deviation and standard error.

Essential Statistics for Bioscientists, First Edition. Mohammed Meah.
© 2022 John Wiley & Sons Ltd. Published 2022 by John Wiley & Sons Ltd.

Experiment: a study of cause and effect. It involves manipulation of one variable (independent variable) while controlling other variables so that they do not affect the outcome, in order to discover the effect on another variable (dependent variable). The independent variable is the one that the experimenter has decided to vary.

Experimental design: the model (control, intervention, protocol) being followed in an experiment which also affects the statistical methods used for the analysis of the results.

Experimental hypothesis: states that there will be a significant difference between conditions. One-stailed hypothesis states that there will be a difference in a specified direction. If its two-tailed, then the direction of the difference is not specified.

Forest plot: combined results plot from many studies investigating the same aim.

Frequency: number of values which are the same in a sample of data.

Frequency distribution curve: a plot of frequency against data (x) or classes of data; distributions can be normal or skewed.

Funnel plot: a plot of study size against effect to assess publication bias.

Histogram: diagram showing the frequency distribution of the data.

Independent variable: variable, which is changed, manipulated in an experiment.

Inferential: analyses sample data to draw conclusions about a population.

Kurtosis: describes how peaked or flat a frequency distribution is.

Mean or average of a sample of data: the sum of the data divided by the number of data.

Median: central or middle number of the data.

Meta-analysis: a statistical method to quantify the results from a systematic review of a specific aim.

Mode: the most frequent value in a sample of data.

Nominal data: data which are characteristic features, e.g., country, gender, colour, ethnicity, religion, and blood type, and which cannot be ordered. The data is qualitative.

Non-parametric tests: statistical tests which do not require the data to be normally distributed. They are less powerful, use nominal and ordinal data, e.g., Wilcoxon's, sign test, Mann–Whitney and Spearman's correlation.

Normal distribution: a frequency distribution curve that has a bell shape with the mean, median, and mode at the same value and the same shape either side of the mean.

Null hypothesis: states that there will be no significant difference between the conditions (usually in the means or medians).

Ogive: cumulative frequency curve.

One-tailed test: test used to look for differences in the mean or median in one direction.

Ordinal data: data which can be ordered or ranked, e.g., position in a race, hardness of materials, level of pain, level of anxiety. The data is qualitative and quantitative.

Outliers: values which are high or low and stand out from the majority of values.

P value: the probability that the result occurred due to chance factors. p<0.05 is significant, p>0.05 is not significant. If p is large, then the result is unreliable, the smaller the value the less likely the result was due to chance.

Parameter: any statistical information taken from a population.

Parametric tests: powerful statistical tests which assume that the data is normally distributed and mainly use continuous data, e.g., t-tests, ANOVA, Pearson's correlation.

Percentile: a term used to describe where a score is in relation to the other data in the sample, e.g., if a score is the 60th percentile, then 60% of the other data are below the score.

Population: the total parts, persons, or groups being investigated or studied, e.g., all employees of a company, population of a country, male students.

Post hoc tests: tests to determine which pairs in an ANOVA test are significant.

Prospective (longitudinal or cohort): study-data collected from cohorts in the future.

Qualitative variables: tend to be characteristics of a population or sample such as gender, ethnicity, and profession.

Quartiles: a measure of the spread of data after dividing them into four intervals (quarters or 25% for each interval).

Random sample: sample chosen in a random manner, each member has an equal chance of being selected.

Range: the difference between the largest value and the smallest value.

Raw data: collected data or observations.

Regression: statistical method to quantify the relationship between two or more variables.

Reliability: a measure of the consistency of a test or measurement after repetition.

Replicates: number of times data is measured again.

Retrospective: study-data collected from the past.

Sample: a part of a population being investigated, usually collected randomly.

Scatter plot: a graph showing data points of two variables.

Significance: if a test tells us that the result was probably not due to chance, the difference is said to be significant.

Significance level: normally taken at the 5% (0.05) level of probability, i.e., there is only a 5% probability (1 in 20) that result occurred due to chance. Others include 1% and 0.1%.

Significant difference: a difference that is unlikely to have occurred by chance.

Skewness: describes the asymmetry or departure from a symmetrical frequency distribution.

Skewed distribution: data distribution is clustered to the left or right usually.

Standard deviation (SD): measure of the distribution of data around the mean.

Standard error of the mean (SEM): a measure of the accuracy of the mean. Mathematically it is the standard deviation divided by the square root of the sample size.

Statistic: any estimate of statistical attribute taken from a sample.

Statistics: deals with collection, organization, presentation, analysis, interpretation of data to obtain meaningful and useful information.

Stratified sample: divide into two groups of similar characteristics, then draw sample from each group.

Student's t distribution: related to the normal distribution and used to compare two groups for significance.

Systematic review: a method of reviewing a subject area by selecting, evaluating, and synthesizing the available literature using defined inclusion and exclusion criteria.

t value: mathematically, this is the mean divided by the standard error of the mean. For a given level of degree of freedom and significance level a significant difference in the means between two groups is shown if the experimental t value is greater than the predicted t value.

t-tests: inferential tests to test for significance between two groups.

Transform: to mathematically convert data so that it approximates to a normal distribution.

Two-tailed test: test used to look for any changes between groups.

Type 1 error: where a result is reported significant when it is not.

Type 2 error: where a result is reported as not significant when it is, commonly occurs if N, the number of data collected for analysis, is low.

Validity: a measure of the accuracy of a test or measurement.

Variable: a specific factor, property, or characteristic of a population or a sample.

Variance: describes how much a random variable differs from its expected value. It is also the square of the standard deviation and is a measure of the distribution of data around the mean.

Z scores: are standard scores which show how far from the mean an individual score falls and can be used to compare an individual's scores on different tests provided they are normally distributed.

Appendix 3

Common Symbols Used in Statistics

Σ (sigma) = summation

CI = confidence interval

d = difference between paired data.

df = degrees of freedom

E = margin of error

f = frequency

F_{crit} = critical value of F

H_1 or H_a = alternative hypothesis

H_o = null hypothesis

HT = hypothesis test

IQR = interquartile range ($Q_3 - Q_1$)

m = slope of a line

M or **Med** = median of a sample

N = population size.

n = sample size, number of data points

p = probability value

$Q1$ = first quartile

$Q3$ = third quartile

r = linear correlation coefficient of a sample

r^2 = coefficient of determination

s = standard deviation of a sample

SD (or s.d.) = standard deviation

SEM = standard error of the mean

t = t value

t_{crit} = critical value of t

$\bar{x}$ (x bar) = mean of a sample

x = one data value

z = standard score or z-score

Essential Statistics for Bioscientists, First Edition. Mohammed Meah.
© 2022 John Wiley & Sons Ltd. Published 2022 by John Wiley & Sons Ltd.

α (alpha) = significance level in hypothesis test

μ (mu) = mean of a population

ρ (rho) = linear correlation coefficient of a population.

σ (sigma) = standard deviation of a population

χ^2 (chi) = chi-squared

Appendix 4

Standard Formulas

1. Arithmetic mean $\bar{x} = \dfrac{\sum x}{n}$

2. Standard deviation (sd) $= \sqrt{\dfrac{\sum (x-\bar{x})^2}{n-1}}$

3. Variance $= sd^2$

4. Variance = sum of squares/degrees of freedom $= \dfrac{\sum (x-\bar{x})^2}{n-1}$

5. Standard error of the mean (SEM) $= \dfrac{sd}{\sqrt{n}}$

6. Coefficient of variation CV (%) = sd x 100/mean

7. Confidence interval (CI) $= \bar{x} \pm t\left(\dfrac{sd}{\sqrt{n}}\right)$

   Where t has n-1 degrees of freedom

8. *Paired t-test*

   t = difference in means/standard error

   $t = \dfrac{\bar{x}-u}{\dfrac{sd}{\sqrt{n}}}$

   degrees of freedom $= n$-1

9. *Unpaired t-test (independent) with equal variances*

   $t = \dfrac{\overline{x1}-\overline{x2}}{sdc\sqrt{\dfrac{1}{n1}+\dfrac{1}{n2}}}$; $sdc = \sqrt{\dfrac{s1^2(n1-1)+s2^2(n2-1)}{(n1+n2-2)}}$

   Degrees of freedom $= n1 + n2$-2; sdc = standard deviation combined; s1 and s2 = standard deviations of sample 1 and 2; $n1$ and $n2$ = sample sizes

10. *Unpaired t-test (independent) with unequal variances*

    $t = \dfrac{\overline{x1}-\overline{x2}}{\sqrt{\dfrac{s1^2}{n1}+\dfrac{s2^2}{n2}}}$

Essential Statistics for Bioscientists, First Edition. Mohammed Meah.
© 2022 John Wiley & Sons Ltd. Published 2022 by John Wiley & Sons Ltd.

11. Correlation coefficient (r)

$$r = \frac{\sum (x - \bar{x})(y - \bar{y})}{(\sum (x - \bar{x})^2 \sum (y - \bar{y})^2)^{0.5}} = -1 \text{ to} + 1$$

12. Z score

Z = (observed value – sample mean)/standard deviation of sample = $(X - \bar{x})$/SD

13. Chi-squared

$X^2 = \sum [(O\text{-}E)/E]$ where, O = observed readings, E = estimated readings

14. Combinations- $nC_r = n!/((n\text{-}r)! \times r!)$
15. Permutations- $nP_r = n!/(n\text{-}r)!$

Appendix 5

How to Calculate Sample Size

There are several methods to calculate sample size depending on the type of study and design. The equations that are used also vary. This is not an easy topic.

Method 1: The difference between sample mean and population mean is an error, called the margin of error (ME).

ME = maximum difference between observed sample mean ($\bar{x}$) and the true population mean (μ).

Or ME = critical value x (SD/$\sqrt{N}$),
Or, N = ((critical value x SD)/ME)^2

Where,

N = sample size we want to find,

SD = population standard deviation (SD), need to estimate this (it is a measure of variation),

Critical value = $Z_{a/2}$

To find N, we need to decide a number of things. For the critical value we need to decide what confidence level to use, most common is the 95% level, so in the formula above we can replace it with 1.96. For the ME, we can decide on an acceptable value such as 5% or more. The last thing we need is the population standard deviation. We would need to research the literature and estimate this for the population we are going to take our sample from.

i.e., $N = ((1.96 \text{ x SD})/0.05)^2$

Method 2: This is very similar to above but is better for larger size studies (Cochrane, 1989). The formula for the sample size is:

N = (Z^2 x SD x (1-SD)/ME^2

Where, Z = critical value, SD = standard deviation, ME = margin of error.

Suppose we chose the following and put them in the formula:
if we choose the 95% confidence level, then Z can be replaced with 1.96, the SD could be estimated as 0.5 and we will set ME at 5%.

Or, N = (1.96^2 x 0.5) x (1-0.5)/ (0.05^2)
Or, N = (3.84 x 0.5) x (0.5)/0.0025
Or, N = (1.92 x 0.5)/0.0025
Or N = 384

Essential Statistics for Bioscientists, First Edition. Mohammed Meah.
© 2022 John Wiley & Sons Ltd. Published 2022 by John Wiley & Sons Ltd.

This is a large sample. To reduce the size, we need to reduce the confidence level or increase the margin of error or both.

There are many other methods, some based on the power of the study required (typically 80%), the effect size, type of statistical test planned (e.g., t-test, ANOVA), but nearly all need standard deviation.

Appendix 6

Familiarisation with GraphPad Prism

Prism is very good for displaying data graphically and for analysis of data. The examples shown in this book have used Prism version 4. If you are using a higher version of Prism, the instructions are going to be different but you will be able to quickly adapt to the newer version formats which have more guidance and help provided in user guides and statistical guidance for tests (available from the website https://www.graphpad.com/scientific-software/prism).

Depending on your version, when you start Prism, you will be shown a welcome page as shown below.

Below is the welcome page for Prism version 4.

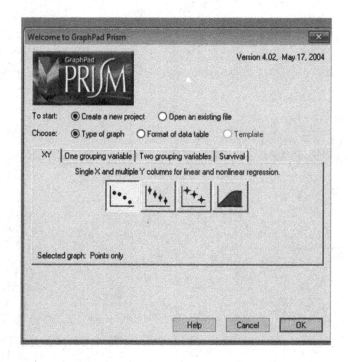

Essential Statistics for Biosciences, First Edition. Mohammed Meah.
© 2022 John Wiley & Sons Ltd. Published 2022 by John Wiley & Sons Ltd.

Below is the welcome page for Prism version 6.

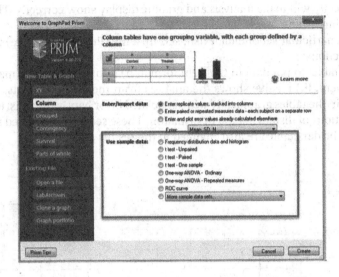

The latest version is Prism 9. Again the welcome dialogue is shown below.

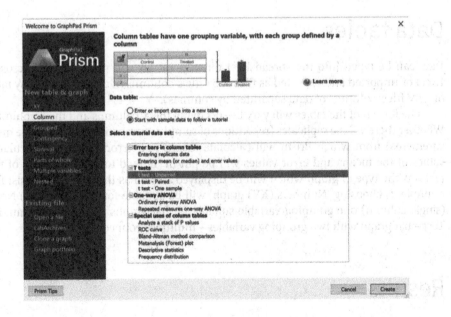

The welcome page allows you to choose how your data will be set up in a data table in the right format. Prism 6 has six formats and Prism 9 has eight formats. Setting this up correctly will make analysis and graphic display show correctly. This formatting is very important.

For any particular set of data, Prism sets up a file (Prism project file) which contains five sections:

i) Data table: to put data in the right format, ii) info: to input information about the experiment, iii) results: shows the analysis from the statistical tests, iv) graphs: shows data in the tables graphically with associated error bars, v) layouts: to show the different options of displaying the information. These sections are linked so that any changes in the data table are also changed in the results and graphs.

Data tables

Data can be typed into the spreadsheet directly, or cut and pasted from Microsoft Excel or imported and exported as files (text files: columns of data separated by tabs; or CSV files: columns of data separated by commas).

The format of the tables will vary by specifying the X columns and the Y columns. Whether there will be replicates (repetitions of samples or repetitions of the same measurements) from which Prism will calculate means and error bars or precalculated values of the means and error values will be put in. Linked to the formatting of the tables is the type of graph which will be displayed as well as the type of analysis. For example: i) choosing 'Numbers (XY) graph' will be suitable for line graphs, ii) None (single column) one grouping variable suitable for bar graphs with no x column, iii) Text – bar graph with two grouping variables – multiple grouped bar graphs.

Results

The 'Analyze' button is used in either the data table or graph section to select built in analysis in prism. You choose the type of analysis and also whether all the data sets or selected data sets are analysed. There is a 'help me decide' button to help with choosing the type of statistical test.

Graphs

Prism automatically sets up one graph from each data table. If data is changed in the data table the analysis and graphs are automatically updated.

Changes

Using the 'New', 'Analyze' and 'Change' buttons you can quickly alter the Prism project file. The 'New' tab allows creation of new sheets, data tables, graphs or layouts. The 'Change' button allows all aspects of graphs to be altered. The options are wide.

Appendix 7

Answers to Sample Problems
Chapter 1

Q1. i) Nominal, ii) Discrete, iii) Ordinal, iv) Continuous, v) Continuous.

Q2.

Mean	Median	Mode	Range	SD	SEM
345.8 g	324 g	300 g	383 g	113.6 g	27.6 g

Q3.

i) 95% Confidence Interval $= \text{mean} \pm t_{value} \times \text{SEM}$

From the raw data, the mean = 4077 μL, SEM= 68.41 μL, N=10, df (degrees of freedom)= N-1 = 9, t_{value} obtained from t table at P=5% or 0.05 and df =9, is 2.262

Substituting into equation:
95% confidence interval $= 4077 \pm (2.262 \times 68.41) = 4077 \pm 154.76$ μL
Or $\qquad\qquad\qquad = 3922.23$ and 4231.77 μL

ii) Coefficient of variation $= (\text{SD/mean}) \times 100$
$\qquad\qquad\qquad\qquad\qquad = (216.35/4077) \times 100$
$\qquad\qquad\qquad\qquad\qquad = 5.31\%$

Chapter 2

Q1.

TABLE 2.6 Skinfold measurements at four sites

Student	Age	Gender	Suprailliac			Subscapula			Biceps			Triceps		
	Yrs		mm	mm	mm	mm	mm	mm	mm	mm	mm	mm	mm	mm
1	18	M	5.2	5.4	5.8	7.1	7.7	8	13.2	2.3	1.8	4.5	5.5	4
2	19	M	7.1	7.8	8.4	6.5	8	7.1	3	4.1	3.5	5.9	4.8	5.6
3	18.5	F	10.4	11	11.9	8.4	8.7	9	5.4	5.7	6	7.8	7.2	7.9
4	21	F	12.3	13.5	15.5	8.5	10.5	9.3	3.2	4.3	4.1	5.8	6.5	7.8
N	4		4	4	4	4	4	4	4	4	4	4	4	4
Mean	19.1		8.8	9.4	10.4	7.6	8.7	8.4	6.2	4.1	3.9	6.0	6.0	6.3
SD	1.3		3.2	3.6	4.2	1.0	1.3	1.0	4.8	1.4	1.7	1.4	1.1	1.9
SEM	0.7		1.6	1.8	2.1	0.5	0.6	0.5	2.4	0.7	0.9	0.7	0.5	0.9

Essential Statistics for Bioscientists, First Edition. Mohammed Meah.
© 2022 John Wiley & Sons Ltd. Published 2022 by John Wiley & Sons Ltd.

Q2. The plot of absorbance against concentration is shown below.

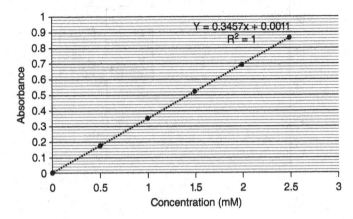

If the absorbance is 0.653, then to find the unknown concentration, we can use the straight line equation for the calibration graph,

i.e., $Y = 0.3457X + 0.0011$

From this equation we can see that the slope $= 0.3457$ and the intercept on the Y axis is 0.0011, Y= absorbance and X= concentration.

Or, $0.653 = 0.3457X + 0.0011$
Or, $0.653-0.0011 = 0.3457X$
Or, $X = (0.653-0.0011)/0.3457$
Or, $X = 1.89$ mM

Q3.

i) Stem and leaf plot

Stem	Leaf
3	0.9
4	0.5
5	
6	0.347
7	0.488
8	0.5

Note, the stem for 5 is still put in, even though there are no data values beginning with 5.

ii) Box Plot
- Median= 6.7
- IQR=2.4
- minute=3.9
- Max=8.5

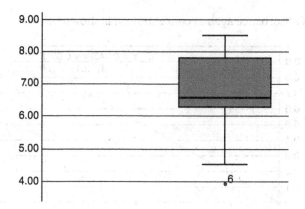

Q4.

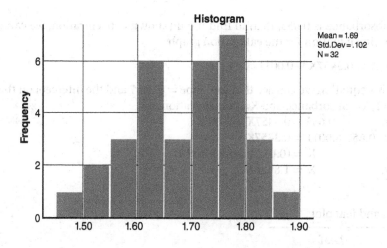

This histogram appears to show an approximate normal distribution. Tests of normality using the Kolmogorov–Smirnov and Shapiro–Wilks tests, showed no significant difference and thus this approximation to normality is accepted.

Q5.

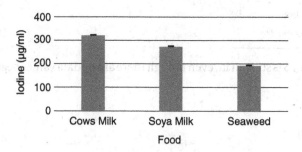

FIGURE 2.32 Mean iodine content ±SEM versus food.

Chapter 3

Q1. In this experiment we have the independent variables as the treatment (antibiotic A and B), and we have the dependent variables, the outcome of being cured or not cured. The number cured for each antibiotic has been given. The question can be tested by using either Fisher's Test or the Chi-squared test.

Q2. Here, nicotine is being measured by an existing standard method and by two other methods. We are not given information on sample size, but do have continuous data and would need to check for normality. As there are more than two comparisons, a one-way ANOVA test would be suitable.

Q3. In this question we have one factor which is the level of diabetes, another factor is the treatment or intervention which is exercise. We have three independent groups. We would choose a two-way ANOVA test to answer the questions about the effect of the diabetes, or the effect of the exercise and any interaction between exercise and diabetes level.

Q4. As the same subject in the control is also being tilted in all the other tilt angles, this would be a repeated measures ANOVA. The data collected is continuous data. There would be more than two comparisons of the mean.

Chapter 4

Q1. A paired t-test was used to compare the means. A significant difference was found between the drug and control (P=0.019). Thus the drug is effective in inducing sleep and the null hypothesis can be rejected.

Q2. A paired t-test was used to compare the means between bronchodilator A and B. No significant difference was found (P=0.062). So, one bronchodilator does not work longer than the other and the null hypothesis is accepted.

Q3. A one-way ANOVA test was used to compare the different antibiotics. A significant difference was found between the four treatments. Post hoc tests (Tukey, Bonferroni) showed that antibiotic D was significantly different from antibiotics A,B and C.

Q4. A correlation test was done between ventilation and heart rate. There was a significant correlation between them. The correlation coefficient showed a high association (r=0.978).

Chapter 5

Q1. A Wilcoxon paired rank analysis was done for the before and after groups, since the sample was not normally distributed. There was no significant difference in the medians, so increased urine flow was not due to the drug.

Q2. From a Mann–Whitney test (not normally distributed, group A was significantly different from group B).

Q3. From a Wilcoxon test, the scores 1 and 2 were not significantly different.

Q4.

Treatment	Improved health	Unchanged health	Totals
Group A (drug)	30	15	45
Group B (placebo)	10	45	55
Totals	40	60	100

Observed (O)	Expected (E)	O-E	$(O-E)^2$	$(O-E)^2/E$
30	45 x (40/100)=18	12	144	8.00
15	45 x (60/100)=27	-12	144	5.33
10	55 x (40/100)=22	-12	144	6.55
45	55 x (60/100)=33	12	144	4.36

Total X^2 =24.242

From the X^2 distribution, for df=1, for $P_{5\%}$ X^2 =3.84

Since 24.2 is > the critical X^2 value of 3.84, drug treatment significantly improves health.

Appendix 8

Standard Critical Tables

i) Z normal, ii) t, iii) F, iv) chi-squared, v) sign, vi) Wilcoxon paired, vii) Mann–Whitney, viii) Pearson correlation coefficients, ix) Spearman's rank.

Cumulative Standardized Normal Distribution

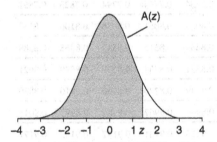

$A(z)$ is the integral of the standardized normal distribution from $-\infty$ to z (in other words, The area under the curve to the left of z). It gives the probability of a normal random variable not being more than z standard deviations above its mean. Values of z of particular importance.

Z	A(z)	
1.645	0.9500	Lower limit of right 5% tail
1.960	0.9750	Lower limit of right 2.5% tail
2.326	0.9900	Lower limit of right 1% tail
2.576	0.9950	Lower limit of right 0.5% tail
3.090	0.9990	Lower limit of right 0.1% tail
3.291	0.9995	Lower limit of right 0.05% tail

Essential Statistics for Bioscientists, First Edition. Mohammed Meah.
© 2022 John Wiley & Sons Ltd. Published 2022 by John Wiley & Sons Ltd.

z	0.00	0.01	0.02	0.03	0.04	0.05	0.06	0.07	0.08	0.09
0.0	0.5000	0.5040	0.5080	0.5120	0.5160	0.5199	0.5239	0.5279	0.5319	0.5359
0.1	0.5398	0.5438	0.5478	0.5517	0.5557	0.5596	0.5636	0.5675	0.5714	0.5753
0.2	0.5793	0.5832	0.5871	0.5910	0.5948	0.5987	0.6026	0.6064	0.6103	0.6141
0.3	0.6179	0.6217	0.6255	0.6293	0.6331	0.6368	0.6406	0.6443	0.6480	0.6517
0.4	0.6554	0.6591	0.6628	0.6664	0.6700	0.6736	0.6772	0.6808	0.6844	0.6879
0.5	0.6915	0.6950	0.6985	0.7019	0.7054	0.7088	0.7123	0.7157	0.7190	0.7224
0.6	0.7257	0.7291	0.7324	0.7357	0.7389	0.7422	0.7454	0.7486	0.7517	0.7549
0.7	0.7580	0.7611	0.7642	0.7673	0.7704	0.7734	0.7764	0.7794	0.7823	0.7852
0.8	0.7881	0.7910	0.7939	0.7967	0.7995	0.8023	0.8051	0.8078	0.8106	0.8133
0.9	0.8159	0.8186	0.8212	0.8238	0.8264	0.8289	0.8315	0.8340	0.8365	0.8389
1.0	0.8413	0.8438	0.8461	0.8485	0.8508	0.8531	0.8554	0.8577	0.8599	0.8621
1.1	0.8643	0.8665	0.8686	0.8708	0.8729	0.8749	0.8770	0.8790	0.8810	0.8830
1.2	0.8849	0.8869	0.8888	0.8907	0.8925	0.8944	0.8962	0.8980	0.8997	0.9015
1.3	0.9032	0.9049	0.9066	0.9082	0.9099	0.9115	0.9131	0.9147	0.9162	0.9177
1.4	0.9192	0.9207	0.9222	0.9236	0.9251	0.9265	0.9279	0.9292	0.9306	0.9319
1.5	0.9332	0.9345	0.9357	0.9370	0.9382	0.9394	0.9406	0.9418	0.9429	0.9441
1.6	0.9452	0.9463	0.9474	0.9484	0.9495	0.9505	0.9515	0.9525	0.9535	0.9545
1.7	0.9554	0.9564	0.9573	0.9582	0.9591	0.9599	0.9608	0.9616	0.9625	0.9633
1.8	0.9641	0.9649	0.9656	0.9664	0.9671	0.9678	0.9686	0.9693	0.9699	0.9706
1.9	0.9713	0.9719	0.9726	0.9732	0.9738	0.9744	0.9750	0.9756	0.9761	0.9767
2.0	0.9772	0.9778	0.9783	0.9788	0.9793	0.9798	0.9803	0.9808	0.9812	0.9817
2.1	0.9821	0.9826	0.9830	0.9834	0.9838	0.9842	0.9846	0.9850	0.9854	0.9857
2.2	0.9861	0.9864	0.9868	0.9871	0.9875	0.9878	0.9881	0.9884	0.9887	0.9890
2.3	0.9893	0.9896	0.9898	0.9901	0.9904	0.9906	0.9909	0.9911	0.9913	0.9916
2.4	0.9918	0.9920	0.9922	0.9925	0.9927	0.9929	0.9931	0.9932	0.9934	0.9936
2.5	0.9938	0.9940	0.9941	0.9943	0.9945	0.9946	0.9948	0.9949	0.9951	0.9952
2.6	0.9953	0.9955	0.9956	0.9957	0.9959	0.9960	0.9961	0.9962	0.9963	0.9964
2.7	0.9965	0.9966	0.9967	0.9968	0.9969	0.9970	0.9971	0.9972	0.9973	0.9974
2.8	0.9974	0.9975	0.9976	0.9977	0.9977	0.9978	0.9979	0.9979	0.9980	0.9981
2.9	0.9981	0.9982	0.9982	0.9983	0.9984	0.9984	0.9985	0.9985	0.9986	0.9986
3.0	0.9987	0.9987	0.9987	0.9988	0.9988	0.9989	0.9989	0.9989	0.9990	0.9990

(Continued)

(Continued)

z	0.00	0.01	0.02	0.03	0.04	0.05	0.06	0.07	0.08	0.09
3.1	0.9990	0.9991	0.9991	0.9991	0.9992	0.9992	0.9992	0.9992	0.9993	0.9993
3.2	0.9993	0.9993	0.9994	0.9994	0.9994	0.9994	0.9994	0.9995	0.9995	0.9995
3.3	0.9995	0.9995	0.9995	0.9996	0.9996	0.9996	0.9996	0.9996	0.9996	0.9997
3.4	0.9997	0.9997	0.9997	0.9997	0.9997	0.9997	0.9997	0.9997	0.9997	0.9998
3.5	0.9998	0.9998	0.9998	0.9998	0.9998	0.9998	0.9998	0.9998	0.9998	0.9998
3.6	0.9998	0.9998	0.9999							

Critical Values of the t Distribution

df	2-tailed testing			1-tailed testing		
	$\alpha = .1$	$\alpha = .05$	$\alpha = .01$	$\alpha = .1$	$\alpha = .05$	$\alpha = .01$
5	2.015	2.571	4.032	1.476	2.015	3.365
6	1.943	2.447	3.707	1.440	1.943	3.143
7	1.895	2.365	3.499	1.415	1.895	2.998
8	1.860	2.306	3.355	1.397	1.860	2.896
9	1.833	2.262	3.250	1.383	1.833	2.821
10	1.812	2.228	3.169	1.372	1.812	2.764
11	1.796	2.201	3.106	1.363	1.796	2.718
12	1.782	2.179	3.055	1.356	1.782	2.681
13	1.771	2.160	3.012	1.350	1.771	2.650
14	1.761	2.145	2.977	1.345	1.761	2.624
15	1.753	2.131	2.921	1.341	1.753	2.602
16	1.746	2.120	2.898	1.337	1.746	2.583
17	1.740	2.110	2.878	1.333	1.740	2.567
18	1.734	2.101	2.878	1.330	1.734	2.552
19	1.729	2.093	2.861	1.328	1.729	2.539
20	1.725	2.086	2.845	1.325	1.725	2.528
21	1.721	2.080	2.831	1.323	1.721	2.518

(Continued)

(Continued)

df	2-tailed testing			1-tailed testing		
	$\alpha = .1$	$\alpha = .05$	$\alpha = .01$	$\alpha = .1$	$\alpha = .05$	$\alpha = .01$
22	1.717	2.074	2.819	1.321	1.717	2.508
23	1.714	2.069	2.807	1.319	1.714	2.500
24	1.711	2.064	2.797	1.318	1.711	2.492
25	1.708	2.060	2.787	1.316	1.708	2.485
26	1.706	2.056	2.779	1.315	1.706	2.479
27	1.703	2.052	2.771	1.314	1.703	2.473
28	1.701	2.048	2.763	1.313	1.701	2.467
29	1.699	2.045	2.756	1.311	1.699	2.462
30	1.697	2.042	2.750	1.310	1.697	2.457
40	1.684	2.021	2.704	1.303	1.684	2.423
50	1.676	2.009	2.678	1.299	1.676	2.403
60	1.671	2.000	2.660	1.296	1.671	2.390
80	1.664	1.990	2.639	1.292	1.664	2.374
100	1.660	1.984	2.626	1.290	1.660	2.364
120	1.658	1.980	2.617	1.289	1.658	2.358
∞	1.645	1.960	2.576	1.282	1.645	2.327

Critical Values of the F Distribution ($\alpha = .05$)

df within	df between										
	1	2	3	4	5	6	7	8	12	24	∞
5	6.61	5.79	5.41	5.19	5.05	4.95	4.88	4.82	4.68	4.53	4.37
6	5.99	5.14	4.76	4.53	4.39	4.28	4.21	4.15	4.00	3.84	3.67
7	5.59	4.74	4.35	4.12	3.97	3.87	3.79	3.73	3.57	3.41	3.23
8	5.32	4.46	4.07	3.84	3.69	3.58	3.50	3.44	3.28	3.12	2.93
9	5.12	4.26	3.86	3.63	3.48	3.37	3.29	3.23	3.07	2.90	2.71
10	4.96	4.10	3.71	3.48	3.33	3.22	3.14	3.07	2.91	2.74	2.54
11	4.84	3.98	3.59	3.36	3.20	3.09	3.01	2.95	2.79	2.61	2.41

(Continued)

(Continued)

df within	df between										
	1	**2**	**3**	**4**	**5**	**6**	**7**	**8**	**12**	**24**	**∞**
12	4.75	3.89	3.49	3.26	3.11	3.00	2.91	2.85	2.69	2.51	2.30
13	4.67	3.81	3.41	3.18	3.03	2.92	2.83	2.77	2.60	2.42	2.21
14	4.60	3.74	3.34	3.11	2.96	2.85	2.76	2.70	2.53	2.35	2.13
15	4.54	3.68	3.29	3.06	2.90	2.79	2.71	2.64	2.48	2.29	2.07
16	4.49	3.63	3.24	3.01	2.85	2.74	2.66	2.59	2.42	2.24	2.01
17	4.45	3.59	3.20	2.96	2.81	2.70	2.61	2.55	2.38	2.19	1.96
18	4.41	3.55	3.16	2.93	2.77	2.66	2.58	2.51	2.34	2.15	1.92
19	4.38	3.52	3.13	2.90	2.74	2.63	2.54	2.48	2.31	2.11	1.88
20	4.35	3.49	3.10	2.87	2.71	2.60	2.51	2.45	2.28	2.08	1.84
21	4.32	3.47	3.07	2.84	2.68	2.57	2.49	2.42	2.25	2.05	1.81
22	4.30	3.44	3.05	2.82	2.66	2.55	2.46	2.40	2.23	2.03	1.78
23	4.28	3.42	3.03	2.80	2.64	2.53	2.44	2.37	2.20	2.01	1.76
24	4.26	3.40	3.01	2.78	2.62	2.51	2.42	2.36	2.18	1.98	1.73
25	4.24	3.39	2.99	2.76	2.60	2.49	2.40	2.34	2.16	1.96	1.71
26	4.23	3.37	2.98	2.74	2.59	2.47	2.39	2.32	2.15	1.95	1.69
27	4.21	3.35	2.96	2.73	2.57	2.46	2.37	2.31	2.13	1.93	1.67
28	4.20	3.34	2.95	2.71	2.56	2.45	2.36	2.29	2.12	1.91	1.66
29	4.18	3.33	2.93	2.70	2.55	2.43	2.35	2.28	2.10	1.90	1.64
30	4.17	3.32	2.92	2.69	2.53	2.42	2.33	2.27	2.09	1.89	1.62
40	4.08	3.23	2.84	2.61	2.45	2.34	2.25	2.18	2.00	1.79	1.51
60	4.00	3.15	2.76	2.53	2.37	2.25	2.17	2.10	1.92	1.70	1.39
80	3.96	3.11	2.72	2.49	2.33	2.21	2.13	2.06	1.88	1.65	1.33
100	3.94	3.09	2.70	2.46	2.31	2.19	2.10	2.03	1.85	1.63	1.28
120	3.92	3.07	2.68	2.45	2.29	2.18	2.09	2.02	1.83	1.61	1.26
∞	3.84	3.00	2.61	2.37	2.22	2.10	2.01	1.94	1.75	1.52	1.00

Critical Values of the x^2 Distribution

df	Area in the Upper Tail					
	0.99	0.95	0.9	0.1	0.05	0.01
1	0.000	0.004	0.016	2.706	3.841	6.635
2	0.020	0.103	0.211	4.605	5.991	9.210
3	0.115	0.352	0.584	6.251	7.815	11.345
4	0.297	0.711	1.064	7.779	9.488	13.277
5	0.554	1.145	1.610	9.236	11.070	15.086
6	0.872	1.635	2.204	10.645	12.592	16.812
7	1.239	2.167	2.833	12.017	14.067	18.475
8	1.646	2.733	3.490	13.362	15.507	20.090
9	2.088	3.325	4.168	14.684	16.919	21.666
10	2.558	3.940	4.865	15.987	18.307	23.209
11	3.053	4.575	5.578	17.275	19.675	24.725
12	3.571	5.226	6.304	18.549	21.026	26.217
13	4.107	5.892	7.042	19.812	22.362	27.688
14	4.660	6.571	7.790	21.064	23.685	29.141
15	5.229	7.261	8.547	22.307	24.996	30.578
16	5.812	7.962	9.312	23.542	26.296	32.000
17	6.408	8.672	10.085	24.769	27.587	33.409
18	7.015	9.390	10.865	25.989	28.869	34.805
19	7.633	10.117	11.651	27.204	30.144	36.191
20	8.260	10.851	12.443	28.412	31.410	37.566
21	8.897	11.591	13.240	29.615	32.671	38.932
22	9.542	12.338	14.041	30.813	33.924	40.289
23	10.196	13.091	14.848	32.007	35.172	41.638
24	10.856	13.848	15.659	33.196	36.415	42.980
25	11.524	14.611	16.473	34.382	37.652	44.314

Critical Values of the Wilcoxon Signed Ranks Test

| n | Two-Tailed Test | | One-Tailed Test | |
	α=.05	α=.01	α=.05	α=.01
5	–	–	0	–
6	0	–	2	–
7	2	–	3	0
8	3	0	5	1
9	5	1	8	3
10	8	3	10	5
11	10	5	13	7
12	13	7	17	9
13	17	9	21	12
14	21	12	25	15
15	25	15	30	19
16	29	19	35	23
17	34	23	41	27
18	40	27	47	32
19	46	32	53	37
20	52	37	60	43
21	58	42	67	49
22	65	48	75	55
23	73	54	83	62
24	81	61	91	69
25	89	68	100	76
26	98	75	110	84
27	107	83	119	92
28	116	91	130	101
29	126	100	140	110
30	137	109	151	120

Critical Values of the Wilcoxon Ranked-Sums Test (Two-Tailed Testing)

n	α	m																	
		3	4	5	6	7	8	9	10	11	12	13	14	15	16	17	18	19	20
3	.05	—	—	6	7	7	8	8	9	9	10	10	11	11	12	12	13	13	14
	.01	—	—	—	—	—	—	6	6	6	7	7	7	8	8	8	8	9	9
4	.05	—	10	11	12	13	14	14	15	16	17	18	19	20	21	21	22	23	24
	.01	—	—	—	10	10	11	11	12	12	13	13	14	15	15	16	16	17	18
5	.05	15	16	17	18	20	21	22	23	24	26	27	28	29	30	32	33	34	35
	.01	—	—	15	16	16	17	18	19	20	21	22	22	23	24	25	26	27	28
6	.05	22	23	24	26	27	29	31	32	34	35	37	38	40	42	43	45	46	48
	.01	—	21	22	23	24	25	26	27	28	30	31	32	33	34	36	37	38	39
7	.05	29	31	33	34	36	38	40	42	44	46	48	50	52	54	56	58	60	62
	.01	—	28	29	31	32	34	35	37	38	40	41	43	44	46	47	49	50	52
8	.05	38	40	42	44	46	49	51	53	55	58	60	62	65	67	70	72	74	77
	.01	—	37	38	40	42	43	45	47	49	51	53	54	56	58	60	62	64	66
9	.05	47	49	52	55	57	60	62	65	68	71	73	76	79	82	84	87	90	93
	.01	45	46	48	50	52	54	56	58	61	63	65	67	69	72	74	76	78	81
10	.05	58	60	63	66	69	72	75	78	81	84	88	91	94	97	100	103	107	110
	.01	55	57	59	61	64	66	68	71	73	76	79	81	84	86	89	92	94	97

n	α	M=11	12	13	14	15	16	17	18	19	20	21	22	23	24	25	26	27	28
11	.05	69	72	75	79	82	85	89	92	96	99	103	106	110	113	117	121	124	128
	0.1	66	68	71	76	79	82	84	87	90	93	96	99	102	105	108	111		114
12	.05	82	85	89	92	96	100	104	107	111	115	119	123	127	131	135	139	143	147
	.01	79	81	84	87	90	93	96	99	102	105	109	112	115	119	122	125	129	132
13	.05	95	99	103	107	111	115	119	124	128	132	136	141	145	150	154	158	163	167
	.01	92	34	98	101	104	108	111	115	118	122	125	129	133	136	140	144	148	151
14	.05	110	114	118	122	127	131	136	141	145	150	155	160	164	169	174	179	183	188
	.01	106	109	112	116	120	123	127	131	135	139	143	147	151	155	159	163	168	172
15	.05	125	130	134	139	144	149	154	159	164	169	174	179	184	190	195	200	205	210
	.01	122	125	128	132	136	140	144	149	153	157	162	166	171	175	180	184	189	193
16	.05	142	147	151	157	162	167	173	178	183	189	195	200	206	211	217	222	228	234
	.01	138	141	145	149	154	158	163	167	172	177	181	186	191	196	201	206	210	215
17	.05	159	164	170	175	181	187	192	198	204	210	216	222	228	234	240	246	252	258
	.01	155	159	163	168	172	177	182	187	192	197	202	207	213	218	223	228	234	239
18	.05	178	183	189	195	201	207	213	219	226	232	238	245	251	257	264	270	277	283
	.01	173	177	182	187	192	197	202	208	213	218	224	229	235	241	246	252	258	263
19	.05	197	203	209	215	222	228	235	242	248	255	262	268	275	282	289	296	303	309
	.01	193	197	202	207	212	218	223	229	235	241	247	253	259	264	271	277	283	283
20	.05	218	224	230	237	244	251	258	265	272	279	286	293	300	308	315	322	329	337
	.01	213	218	223	228	234	240	246	252	258	264	270	277	283	289	296	302	309	315

Note: n is the number of scores in the group with the smallest sum of ranks; M is the number of scores in the other group.

Critical Values of the Mann-Whitney U (Two-Tailed Testing)

Columns are n_1.

n_2	α	3	4	5	6	7	8	9	10	11	12	13	14	15	16	17	18	19	20
3	.05	—	—	0	1	1	2	2	3	3	4	4	5	5	6	6	7	7	8
	.01	—	—	—	—	—	—	0	0	0	1	1	1	2	2	2	2	3	3
4	.05		0	1	2	3	4	4	5	6	7	8	9	10	11	11	12	13	14
	.01		—	—	0	0	1	1	2	2	3	3	4	5	5	6	6	7	8
5	.05			2	3	5	6	7	8	9	11	12	13	14	15	17	18	19	20
	.01			0	1	1	2	3	4	5	6	7	7	8	9	10	11	12	13
6	.05				5	6	8	10	11	13	14	16	17	19	21	22	24	25	27
	.01				2	3	4	5	6	7	9	10	11	12	13	15	16	17	18
7	.05					8	10	12	14	16	18	20	22	24	26	28	30	32	34
	.01					4	6	7	9	10	12	13	15	16	18	19	21	22	24
8	.05						13	15	17	19	22	24	26	29	31	34	36	38	41
	.01						7	9	11	13	15	17	18	20	22	24	26	28	30
9	.05							17	20	23	26	28	31	34	37	39	42	45	48
	.01							11	13	16	18	20	22	24	27	29	31	33	36
10	.05								23	26	29	33	36	39	42	45	48	52	55
	.01								16	18	21	24	26	29	31	34	37	39	42

		11	12	13	14	15	16	17	18	19	20
11	.05	30	33	37	40	44	47	51	55	58	62
	.01	21	24	27	30	33	36	39	42	45	48
12	.05		37	41	45	49	53	57	61	65	69
	.01		27	31	34	37	41	44	47	51	54
13	.05			45	50	54	59	63	67	72	76
	.01			34	38	42	45	49	53	57	60
14	.05				55	59	64	69	74	78	83
	.01				42	46	50	54	58	63	67
15	.05					64	70	75	80	85	90
	.01					51	55	60	64	69	73
16	.05						75	81	86	92	98
	.01						60	65	70	74	79
17	.05							87	93	99	105
	.01							70	75	81	86
18	.05								99	106	112
	.01								81	87	92
19	.05									113	119
	.01									93	99
20	.05										127
	.01										105

Pearson's correlation coefficients
Critical Values of r

n	2-tailed testing			1-tailed testing		
	$\alpha = .1$	$\alpha = .05$	$\alpha = .01$	$\alpha = .1$	$\alpha = .05$	$\alpha = .01$
5	0.805	0.878	0.959	0.687	0.805	0.934
6	0.729	0.811	0.917	0.608	0.729	0.882
7	0.669	0.754	0.875	0.551	0.669	0.833
8	0.621	0.707	0.834	0.507	0.621	0.789
9	0.582	0.666	0.798	0.472	0.582	0.750
10	0.549	0.632	0.765	0.443	0.549	0.715
11	0.521	0.602	0.735	0.419	0.521	0.685
12	0.497	0.576	0.708	0.398	0.497	0.658
13	0.476	0.553	0.684	0.380	0.476	0.634
14	0.458	0.532	0.661	0.365	0.458	0.612
15	0.441	0.514	0.641	0.351	0.441	0.592
16	0.426	0.497	0.623	0.338	0.426	0.574
17	0.412	0.482	0.606	0.327	0.412	0.558
18	0.400	0.468	0.590	0.317	0.400	0.543
19	0.389	0.456	0.575	0.308	0.389	0.529
20	0.378	0.444	0.561	0.299	0.378	0.516
21	0.369	0.433	0.549	0.291	0.369	0.503
22	0.360	0.423	0.537	0.284	0.360	0.492
23	0.352	0.413	0.526	0.277	0.352	0.482
24	0.344	0.404	0.515	0.271	0.344	0.472
25	0.337	0.396	0.505	0.265	0.337	0.462
26	0.330	0.388	0.496	0.260	0.330	0.453
27	0.323	0.381	0.487	0.255	0.323	0.445
28	0.317	0.374	0.479	0.250	0.317	0.437
29	0.311	0.367	0.471	0.245	0.306	0.430
30	0.306	0.361	0.463	0.241	0.306	0.423
40	0.264	0.312	0.403	0.207	0.264	0.367
50	0.235	0.279	0.361	0.184	0.235	0.328

(Continued)

(Continued)

n	2-tailed testing			1-tailed testing		
	$\alpha = .1$	$\alpha = .05$	$\alpha = .01$	$\alpha = .1$	$\alpha = .05$	$\alpha = .01$
60	0.214	0.254	0.330	0.168	0.214	0.300
80	0.185	0.220	0.286	0.145	0.185	0.260
100	0.165	0.197	0.256	0.129	0.165	0.232
120	0.151	0.179	0.234	0.118	0.151	0.212
140	0.140	0.166	0.217	0.109	0.140	0.196
160	0.130	0.155	0.203	0.102	0.130	0.184
180	0.123	0.146	0.192	0.096	0.123	0.173
200	0.117	0.139	0.182	0.091	0.117	0.164
300	0.095	0.113	0.149	0.074	0.095	0.134
400	0.082	0.098	0.129	0.064	0.082	0.116
500	0.074	0.088	0.115	0.057	0.074	0.104

Critical Values of Spearman's r

n	2-tailed testing			1-tailed testing		
	α			α		
	.1	.05	.01	.1	.05	.01
5	0.900	1.000	–	0.800	0.900	1.000
6	0.829	0.886	1.000	0.657	0.829	0.943
7	0.714	0.786	0.929	0.571	0.714	0.893
8	0.643	0.738	0.881	0.524	0.643	0.833
9	0.600	0.700	0.833	0.483	0.600	0.783
10	0.564	0.648	0.794	0.455	0.564	0.745
11	0.527	0.609	0.755	0.418	0.527	0.700
12	0.497	0.580	0.727	0.399	0.497	0.671
13	0.478	0.555	0.698	0.379	0.478	0.643
14	0.459	0.534	0.675	0.363	0.459	0.622
15	0.443	0.518	0.654	0.350	0.443	0.600

(Continued)

(Continued)

n	2-tailed testing α			1-tailed testing α		
	.1	.05	.01	.1	.05	.01
16	0.426	0.500	0.632	0.338	0.426	0.582
17	0.412	0.485	0.615	0.326	0.412	0.564
18	0.399	0.470	0.598	0.315	0.399	0.548
19	0.389	0.458	0.582	0.307	0.389	0.533
20	0.379	0.445	0.568	0.298	0.379	0.520
21	0.369	0.435	0.555	0.291	0.369	0.508
22	0.360	0.424	0.543	0.283	0.360	0.496
23	0.352	0.415	0.531	0.277	0.352	0.485
24	0.343	0.406	0.520	0.270	0.343	0.475
25	0.336	0.397	0.510	0.265	0.336	0.465
26	0.330	0.389	0.500	0.259	0.330	0.456
27	0.324	0.382	0.491	0.254	0.324	0.448
28	0.317	0.375	0.483	0.249	0.317	0.440
29	0.311	0.368	0.474	0.244	0.311	0.432
30	0.306	0.362	0.467	0.240	0.306	0.425
32	0.296	0.350	0.452	0.232	0.296	0.411
34	0.287	0.339	0.439	0.225	0.287	0.399
36	0.279	0.330	0.427	0.218	0.279	0.388
38	0.271	0.321	0.415	0.212	0.271	0.378
40	0.264	0.313	0.405	0.207	0.264	0.368
42	0.257	0.305	0.395	0.201	0.257	0.359
44	0.251	0.298	0.386	0.197	0.251	0.351
46	0.246	0.291	0.378	0.192	0.246	0.343
48	0.240	0.285	0.370	0.188	0.240	0.336
50	0.235	0.279	0.363	0.184	0.235	0.329
60	0.214	0.254	0.331	0.168	0.214	0.300
70	0.198	0.235	0.307	0.155	0.198	0.278
80	0.185	0.220	0.287	0.145	0.185	0.260

References

Bjordal, J.M., Ljunggren, A.E., Klovning, A. and Slørdal, L. (2004). Non-steroidal anti-inflammatory drugs, including cyclo-oxygenase-2 inhibitors, in osteoarthritic knee pain: meta-analysis of randomised placebo controlled trials. *The BMJ* 329: 1317.

Bland, J.M. and Altman, D.G. (1986). Statistical methods for assessing agreement between two methods of clinical measurement. *The Lancet*. 327: 307–310.

Bland, J.M. (2009). Analysis of continuous data from small samples. *The BMJ* 338: a3166.

De Winter, J.C.F. (2013). Using the Student's t-test with extremely small sample sizes. *Practical Assessment, Research, and Evaluation* 18: Article 10.

Doll, R. and Hill, A.B. (1950). Smoking and carcinoma of the lung; preliminary report. *The BMJ* 2: 739–748.

D'Souza, A.L., Rajkumar, C., Cooke, J. and Bulpitt, C.J. (2002). Probiotics in prevention of antibiotic associated diarrhoea: meta-analysis. *The BMJ* 324: 1361.

Parkes, M., Cook, A.R., Lim, J.T., Sun, Y. and Dickens, B.L. (2020). A systematic review of COVID-19 epidemiology based on current evidence. *Journal of Clinical Medicine* 9: 967–979.

Wright, R.W., Brand, R.A., Dunn, W. and Spindler, K.P. (2007). How to write a systematic review. *Clinical Orthopaedics And Relate Research* 455: 23–29.

Further Reading

Akobeng, A.K. (2005). Understanding systematic reviews and meta-analysis. *Archives of Disease in Childhood* 90: 845–848.

Ashcroft, S. and Pereira, C. (2003). *Practical Statistics for the Biological Sciences*. Palgrave Macmillan.

Bland, M. (1997). *An Introduction to Medical Statistics*. Oxford Medical Publications.

Blann, A. (2015). *Data Handling and Analysis*. Oxford University Press.

Cochrane, W.G. (1989). *Statistical Methods*. Blackwell.

Dawson-Saunders, B. and Trapp, R.G. (1994). *Basic and Clinical Biostatistics*, 2e. Appleton and Lange.

Dancey, C.P. and Reidy, J. (2001). *Statistics without Maths for Psychology: Using SPSS for Windows*, 2e. London: Prentice Hall.

Dewhurst, F. (2002). *Quantitative Methods for Business and Management*. McGraw Hill Education.

Ennos, R. (2000). *Statistical and Data Handling Skills in Biology*. Pearson Prentice Hall.

Ennos, R. (2007). *Statistical and Data Handling Skills in Biology*. Pearson Prentice Hall.

Heyes, S., Hardy, M., Humphreys, P. and Rookes, P. (1990). *Starting Statistics in Psychology and Education*. Weidenfeld and Nicolson.

Kirkpatrick, L.A. and Feeney, B.C. (2001). *A Simple Guide to SPSS for Windows (Versions 8,9,10)*. Wadsworth.

Kinnear, P.R. and Gray, C.D. (2000). *SPSS for Windows Made Simple: Release 10*. Hove: Psychology Press.

Mahmood, S.S., Levy, D., Vasan, R.S. and Wang, T.J. (2014). The Framingham heart study and the epidemiology of cardiovascular disease: a historical perspective. *The Lancet* 383: 999–1008.

Essential Statistics for Bioscientists, First Edition. Mohammed Meah.
© 2022 John Wiley & Sons Ltd. Published 2022 by John Wiley & Sons Ltd.

Meah, M.S. and Kabedi-Westhead, E. (2012). *Essential Laboratory Skills for Biosciences*. Wiley-Blackwell.

Miller, J.R. (2003). *Graphpad Prism Version 4, Step-by-Step Examples*. San Diego, CA: Graphpad Software inc.

Phoenix, D. (1997). *Introductory Mathematics for the Life Sciences*. Taylor and Francis.

Pontes, E.A.S. (2018). A brief historical overview of the Gaussian curve: From Abraham De Moivre to Johann Carl Friedrich Gauss. *International Journal of Engineering Science Invention* 7 (6): 28–34.

Jones, A., Read, R. and Weyers, J. (2003). *Practical Skills in Biology*, 3e. Pearson Education.

Sokal, R.R. and Rohlf, F.J. (1994). *Biometry*, 3e. W.H.Freeman.

Swinscow, T.D.V. (1996). *Statistics at Square One*, 9e. BMJ.

Tan, S.H. and Tan, S.B. (2010). The correct interpretation of confidence intervals. *Proceedings of Singapore Healthcare* 19 (3): 276–278.

Thomas, E. (2004). An introduction to medical statistics for health care professionals: describing and presenting data. *Musculoskeletal Care* 2 (4): 218–228.

Voysey, M. et al (2021). Safety and efficacy of the ChAdOx1 nCoV-19 vaccine (AZD1222) against SARS-CoV-2: an interim analysis of four randomised controlled trials in Brazil, South Africa, and the UK. *The Lancet* 397: 99–111.

Wakefield, A.J., Murch, S.H., Anthony, A., Linnell, J., Casson, D.M., Malik, M., Berelowitz, M., Dhillon, A.P., Thomson, M.A., Harvey, P., Valentine, A., Davies, S.E. and Walker-Smith, J.A. (1998). Ileal-lymphoid-nodular hyperplasia, non-specific colitis, and pervasive developmental disorder in children. *The Lancet* 351 (9103): 637–641.

Walker, E., Hernandez, A.V. and Kattan, M.W. (2008). Meta-analysis: its strengths and limitations. *Cleveland Clinic Journal of Medicine* 75 (6): 431–439.

Winters, R., Winters, A. and Amedee, R.G. (2010). Statistics: a brief overview. *The Ochsner Journal* 10: 213–216.

Index

Essential Statistics for Bioscientists, First Edition. Mohammed Meah.
© 2022 John Wiley & Sons Ltd. Published 2022 by John Wiley & Sons Ltd.